Fasting Secrets for Chronic Conditions

Proven Strategies to Reset the Immune System, Manage Chronic Inflammation, Optimize Blood Sugar Control, and Feel Better Again

Tina Shelton

direct or indirect, that are incurred as a result of the use of the information contained within this document, including, but not limited to, errors, omissions, or inaccuracies.

Table of Contents

Introduction

When something bad happens, you have three choices. You either let it define you, let it destroy you, or you can let it strengthen you.
–Dr Seuss.

Chronic diseases are something that many people struggle with, and they can cause severe health problems and significantly affect your quality of life. Chronic diseases also severely impact your mental health, and they can cause a lot of tension and distress in your home and family life. To make matters worse, many people are told that their chronic diseases are their fault. They are told that poor lifestyle choices, genetics, and diet cause it. Then, they are also told that there is nothing to do about their chronic disease, that they are resigned to their fate and must suffer in silence while their bodies deteriorate and fail.

But that is not true at all! There are many causes for chronic diseases; genetics, lifestyle choices, and diet and lack of exercise are just some of them. But there are also many cures for chronic diseases. In fact, most chronic diseases, even the most aggressive ones, can be treated and managed with great success. This book will explore some of the alternative therapies available for treating, managing, and overcoming chronic disease. Fasting, specifically prolonged fasting, has effectively treated and managed several chronic conditions, including cancer, heart disease, diabetes, stroke and brain health, IBS, arthritis, and more. And I think it's high time you learn how to incorporate fasting and other lifestyle changes to help you overcome your chronic disease once and for all.

You can feel good about yourself without being heavily medicated. You can have your smile back and feel comfortable in your body all the time. You can fully enjoy life again by using simple fasting tips you will learn in this book. Like many others, chronic diseases have affected my family as well.

I lost my dear dad in 2020 due to prostate cancer, and 4 years earlier, my beloved brother passed away, aged only 31, from a stroke. The pain that resulted from these losses led me to investigate chronic diseases thoroughly, just to find out my dad and brother could have still been with us if they had embarked on some form of fasting lifestyle. Knowledge is power, and that power saves lives.

This book will explore the use of prolonged fasting and other fasting models for improved health and the treatment of chronic diseases. We will explore what fasting is and how it works; how to undertake prolonged fasting safely; what the side effects of fasting are and how to avoid them; and what science says about fasting and chronic disease. We'll explore the works of many brilliant minds and how they have used fasting protocols to help thousands worldwide overcome their chronic diseases. In addition, we will share case studies and success stories you wouldn't believe, to prove how effective fasting is for curing chronic disease—even the most aggressive types of cancer. Furthermore, we will explore how scientific studies back all these claims and success stories to show that prolonged fasting is not just a theory but a valid medical therapy.

If you have been struggling with a chronic disease and conventional therapies aren't working, this book is for you! Whether you want to prevent, treat, or cure a chronic disease, fasting is the way to do it. This book will equip you with all the information you need to take your health to the next level and overcome your chronic disease. By the end of this book, you will have everything you need to make the necessary lifestyle changes and significantly improve your health and well-being. Before we begin, I have one question to ask you. Are you ready to transform your life and beat your chronic disease? Then, let's get started!

Chapter 1:

A Body Without Chronic Disease—An Overview

Chronic diseases can upend your entire life. They cause many problems and may interrupt your daily activities. Therefore, striving for a life free from chronic diseases is something we should all aim for. But if you have been battling chronic disease for some time, you may not know what a body without it feels like. To help you understand what it feels like to live free of chronic disease and to give you the motivation to strive for a life like this, we will discuss what a body without chronic disease feels like. We'll also consider what a body without chronic disease looks like and discuss the anatomy of such a body. Are you ready to learn what you will work towards in this book? Then let's go!

What Does a Body Without Chronic Disease Feel Like?

A chronic disease puts a lot of strain on your body. It means that your body is not functioning optimally, and that will ultimately affect how you feel. You may already know that you don't feel your best when you are chronically ill. But if you have been this way for some time now, you may have forgotten what it feels like to have a healthy body and live without chronic disease. You may have accepted your fate and thought you must feel the way you do. But that is not the case, as you will see in this book. So before we begin with the science behind fasting and curing chronic conditions, I would first like to remind you of what you have to look forward to when you no longer have a chronic disease.

What does a body without chronic disease feel like? Some people reading this book have been living with chronic disease for so long that they no longer know how it feels to live a "normal" and healthy life. To help you remember what a healthy body feels like and give you some much-needed motivation for putting your health first and ending your chronic diseases, I thought it would be wise to share what a body without chronic disease feels like. A healthy body functions optimally. One that uses the energy it gets from the food it receives to empower you to do physically and mentally challenging things.

A healthy body, or one that is free from chronic disease, feels energized, powerful, and comfortable. This body does not feel pain or discomfort when performing any tasks. It also does not get tired easily. Instead, a healthy body free from chronic disease has plenty of stamina and endurance. This body wakes up feeling energized and ready to take on the world. It does not suffer from stiff muscles or joints when it wakes up, and it does not feel drained of energy just after waking up in the morning. A body free from chronic disease is also responsive. Unlike bodies with chronic diseases that sometimes feel a bit lagging, it will do what you tell it to and when you tell it to.

A body without chronic disease feels strong, making you feel confident. There is a strong correlation between mental and physical health. If you have a chronic disease that leads to feeling weak, tired, or unproductive, it will likely affect your confidence. Instead of feeling capable of completing physically and mentally challenging tasks, you will feel like you have no energy. But if you don't have any chronic conditions, you will wake up feeling your best self and feel like you can conquer the world. Therefore, a body without chronic disease will be more responsive and alert than one with it.

Many chronic diseases also lead to brain fog. Therefore, if you have a chronic disease, you may feel slow or sluggish sometimes, especially when the disease flares up. But someone who does not suffer from a chronic disease typically feels clear-headed. This positively impacts their decision-making and problem-solving skills, making them a more valuable asset at work and home. Therefore, people who don't suffer from chronic diseases are typically better employees and make better leaders at work, as their mental capacity and clarity are not hindered by their disease.

All of these aspects affect how healthy people think of themselves. They are willing to take on more work, challenge themselves, and put in the work required to improve themselves in all life aspects. They often have the energy to make time for exercise and healthy lifestyle choices. This also affects their self-esteem and self-confidence. If you can heal your chronic condition, you will have an even greater advantage than people who never had a chronic condition, as you know how much better you feel and how much more you can do now that your health is restored. Your confidence is also greatly affected by your physical appearance. So how does a body without chronic disease look, and how will a healthy body impact your appearance?

What Does a Body Without Chronic Disease Look Like?

Your physical appearance is greatly affected by your health. If you are healthy, your body can manage your energy levels better. You will also sleep better and have more energy during the day. And your immune system is stronger, meaning you won't get sick as often. Therefore, a body without chronic disease typically looks healthier and more vibrant than one with it. But what does a healthy body look like? A healthy body will have the following qualities:

- **Normal blood pressure**—Having normal blood pressure (systolic pressure less than 120 and diastolic pressure less than 80) means your heart is not working too hard to pump blood through your body. It is a sign of a healthy heart and a healthy body.

- **Normal blood sugar levels**—Normal blood sugar levels are between 70 and 100 mg/dL. That means your endocrine system is in good working order and can metabolize the foods you eat effectively without raising your blood sugar levels.

- **Normal cholesterol levels**—High cholesterol is a sign of poor health and can lead to many health conditions, many of which are even worse if you already suffer from chronic disease. There are two types of cholesterol: HDL and LDL. HDL is typically known as "good cholesterol," while LDL is known as "bad cholesterol." Normal cholesterol levels (LDL below 130 mg/dL) mean you are healthy.

- **Strong immune system**—A healthy body has a strong immune system. It won't get sick as often and will fight off bacteria and viruses effectively. You are less likely to get severely sick and more likely to recover faster if you have a strong immune system.

- **Healthy weight**—If your blood pressure, blood sugar, and cholesterol levels are normal, you are more likely also to have a healthy weight since your body can effectively use the energy you provide by eating. Having a healthy weight also increases your overall health and well-being. Your ideal weight is often determined with a body mass index (BMI), a chart that shows your healthy weight based on your height and current weight. A healthy BMI is usually between 18.5 and 24.9. Anything below 18.5 is considered underweight, while a reading higher than 24.9 indicates that you are overweight.

- **Good mental health**—If you are physically healthy, you will also be mentally healthy. Good mental health is crucial for overall well-being, and it is something that is often affected by chronic conditions.

Having a healthy body does not simply happen. Even when you don't have chronic diseases, you still have to work to keep your body healthy and in shape. Doing so requires time and dedication. You can maintain a healthy body by practicing the following habits.

- **Regular physical activity**—150 minutes of weekly training can help you maintain a healthy weight and optimal blood pressure levels.

- **Balanced diet**—A balanced diet is crucial for normal blood sugar levels, healthy weight, and a strong immune system. When you eat is also important as it affects your energy levels throughout the day.

- **Good sleep habits**—Sleep is often overlooked when trying to improve health. Yet studies have shown just how important sleep is for your health and well-being. Getting 7 to 8 hours of sleep daily is crucial for optimal health.

- **Regular health screenings**—If you go for regular health checkups and screenings, you are likelier to detect a problem when it is in its early stages. You can address it sooner and prevent it from becoming a serious health concern.

A Brief Anatomy of a Body Without Chronic Disease

A healthy body is healthy overall. A healthy body will function optimally from a general to a cellular level. Cellular health and organ health are two important aspects of overall health. According to Next Health, "You can think of cellular health as the microscopic version of overall health. The healthier your cells are, the healthier your body should be in aggregate since your cells will work properly and well with one another" (*Cellular Health,* 2023). Your cells are the smallest parts of your body. And when these cells work together, they will ensure all your bodily systems, including your organs and brain, also function optimally. If your cells are healthy, they will ensure that these systems, among others, are also healthy.

Immune System

Your immune system is crucial for keeping you healthy and fighting against diseases. Since some chronic conditions arise from bacteria and viruses, a healthy immune system can also prevent chronic disease.

Cardiovascular System

If your cardiovascular system suffers, so too does your overall health. If your heart is healthy, it can effectively pump oxygen-rich blood to your body and keep your other organs and tissue healthy.

Respiratory System

Without a properly functioning respiratory system, your body will not get the oxygen needed to be healthy. Your respiratory system is crucial for overall health.

Digestive System

Your digestive system is responsible for managing how well your body absorbs nutrients from food. Therefore, if your digestive system does not work properly, your body won't get the nutrients it needs.

Musculoskeletal System

Your musculoskeletal system is responsible for ensuring mobility, strength, and movement. If this system does not function properly, your movement will be affected. Keeping your muscles and skeleton strong and healthy will improve your overall health and well-being.

Nervous System

Your nervous system affects many aspects of your body, including your response to stress and physical stimuli. If your nervous system does not function properly, you may have trouble with movement, coping with stress, and physical stimuli, such as heat and pain.

Endocrine System

Your endocrine system is responsible for many functions and systems throughout your body. It regulates and manages these systems through different hormones. If your endocrine system is compromised, you may have hormonal imbalances, which can cause various health problems.

Reproductive System

The reproductive system is mainly managed through hormones. However, the reproductive system is responsible for more than just reproduction. It also affects weight management, blood glucose levels, and sexual desire. You may notice various changes and health conditions if your reproductive system does not function optimally.

Integumentary System

Your integumentary system comprises your skin, nails, hair, and glands. If this system is compromised, germs and other pathogens may enter your body through your skin, and you may suffer various illnesses as a result. Your skin, hair, and nails will also suffer and become dry, brittle, or flaky.

As you can see, a healthy body without chronic disease functions optimally in many ways. And having a chronic disease can impact your health in more ways than one. But with the right lifestyle changes and diet, you can reverse your chronic disease and live a healthy and fulfilled life.

Key Takeaway From Chapter 1

A body without chronic disease typically feels energetic, comfortable, and free from persistent pain or discomfort. A body without chronic disease is functioning optimally and free from long-term illnesses or conditions. If your body is healthy on a cellular level, you will experience greater overall health. The immune, reproductive, endocrine, cardiovascular, and respiratory systems are some of the systems that determine your overall health and well-being.

Chapter 2:

Chronic Diseases

Since this book deals with how fasting can reduce chronic conditions, and in some cases heal them, it is worth understanding what exactly a chronic condition is. Even if you are living with a chronic condition, you may not know exactly how your condition came to be. And if you are uncertain of what chronic conditions are, it might be useful to learn about some chronic conditions to help you determine if what you have is, in fact, a chronic condition. In this chapter, we will discuss what chronic diseases are and how they develop. We will also consider some common types of chronic conditions.

It's important to remember that the chronic conditions we discuss in this chapter are not an exhaustive list by any means. Instead, you should merely see these conditions as some common examples. The description of chronic diseases discussed in this chapter will give you a much better understanding of what chronic diseases are and if you suffer from one. So, what are chronic diseases, and how do they arise?

Chronic Diseases: What Are They and How Do They Develop?

The definition of chronic disease is somewhat disputed. However, scientists generally agree on defining a chronic disease in terms of how long it lasts, how long the recovery time is, and if it is recurring. So, the generally accepted explanation for a chronic disease is that it lasts for three months or more, has a slow progression and recovery time, and is often recurring. Furthermore, there are several characteristics of chronic diseases. Understanding these can help you determine if you, in fact, have a chronic disease and what could be contributing to the severity and presence of that disease. The characteristics often associated with chronic conditions include:

Complex Causes

Chronic conditions often have complex causes that cannot be identified as easily as others. For example, while it's easy to say that you got the stomach flu from your coworkers as they had it, it's not as easy to pinpoint when and where you may have been exposed to the virus or bacteria that caused your chronic condition. Because it is more difficult to determine the cause of a chronic condition, the treatment plan is also often affected and may vary depending on the suspected cause. Also, given the extended period you are sick for and how long it takes for the disease to affect your health, the cause may be even more complex to determine.

Risk Factors

Chronic conditions also have several complex risk factors. These factors can vary from lifestyle choices, such as diet and bad habits, to genetics, pollutants, and more. The risk factors for different chronic conditions also differ. For example, the risk factors for chronic heart conditions might differ from those for certain types of cancer. On the contrary, other risk factors, such as smoking, may be universal for any chronic condition. Depending on the chronic condition you have, certain lifestyle choices may be a bigger risk factor than others.

Extended Latency Periods

Chronic conditions are also typically connected to extended latency periods. This means it might take a long time for the virus or bacteria to affect your health. For example, you can contract the herpes virus months or even years before having a cold sore or showing any signs of infection. And once you show your first symptoms, it will take some time to "heal" from the disease or infection. Most chronic conditions take a while to start affecting your health, and it also takes some time for the symptoms to disappear once they have appeared.

Long Illnesses in General

Chronic conditions tend to have a longer infection period. This means you typically show symptoms longer if you suffer from a chronic condition than an acute one. While the flu will come and go within a week, chronic conditions can take a few months or even a year or more to heal. This means you may show symptoms of a chronic condition for a long time. It also means that a chronic condition can affect your health, well-being, and lifestyle much longer than an acute condition.

Functional Impairment

While this isn't true for all chronic conditions, many tend to affect your day-to-day life. They might lead to functional impairment or disability. For example, certain chronic conditions might affect your well-being to the extent that you are bedridden for days or weeks. The severity of the functional impairment depends on the chronic condition and how severe your diagnosis is. The treatment's effectiveness will also differ depending on the severity of your condition.

Chronic conditions are also typically identified by how easy they are to cure. While some chronic conditions can be cured entirely, others are life-long, and only the symptoms of the condition can be managed or treated. Fortunately, you can treat many chronic conditions with lifestyle and dietary changes, such as fasting. Your body and natural immune system generally cannot fight off a chronic condition as effectively as in certain acute conditions, such as colds. Instead, most chronic conditions require medical intervention.

While some chronic conditions, such as heart disease, may be life-threatening and require immediate medical attention, other chronic conditions, such as arthritis, are not curable but are unlikely to cause your death. The symptoms of these conditions can be managed, but you will likely have this condition for the rest of your life. Other chronic conditions, like diabetes, are lifelong and require intensive and ongoing medical treatment. If these conditions are not treated, they can prove fatal.

Even though the outlook of chronic conditions is generally pretty bleak, it doesn't have to determine how you will live the rest of your life. After all, this book is written to help you live a normal and fulfilling life with chronic conditions. But what are some of the most common types of chronic disease? Let's consider a few examples to better understand chronic conditions and how they might affect your life.

Common Types of Chronic Disease: An Overview

While there are many chronic diseases—too many to list in one book—there are a few you may have had prior interaction with. Whether you or someone you know have or have had one of these chronic diseases, you will likely have some idea of how they affect your life. Let us discuss three of the most common chronic diseases and how they occur.

Cancer and Other Tumors

Cancer is one of the most common and well-known chronic diseases. According to the *World Cancer Research Fund International*, "There were an estimated 18.1 million cancer cases around the world in 2020. Of these, 9.3 million cases were in men and 8.8 million in women" (Worldwide Cancer Data, n.d.). Some of the most common cancers include breast, lung, colorectal, prostate, stomach, and liver cancer. Non-cancerous (benign) tumors are also common and can occur in many parts of the body, including the sex organs, stomach, and lymph nodes. Genetics, lifestyle choices, and pollutants cause cancers and tumors.

Heart Disease and Stroke

Heart disease and stroke is another common chronic disease. Heart disease is often the result of genetics and lifestyle choices. Many kinds of heart diseases include angina, heart attacks, congenital heart diseases, and heart failure. High blood pressure is a common cause of heart disease and strokes. Strokes occur when a blood clot or sediment blocks the arteries in your brain, depriving the brain of oxygen. Strokes often have long-term consequences, such as weakness, paralysis, memory loss, and personality changes. Heart diseases and strokes have many similar causes. Fortunately, you can reduce your chance of developing certain heart diseases or strokes by making a few lifestyle changes.

Diabetes (and Kidney Health)

Diabetes is another common chronic disease. There are various kinds of diabetes, including gestational, type 1, and type 2 diabetes. Each type of diabetes has a different cause, from pregnancy to diet and lifestyle choices. If diabetes is not managed correctly, it can lead to many subsequent health conditions, including kidney failure. Some types of diabetes, like type 2 diabetes, are curable. Other kinds of diabetes are not curable and must be managed with medication and lifestyle changes. Kidney disease is sometimes curable, depending on its severity. If the kidney disease has developed too far, it can only be treated with a kidney replacement.

Risk Factors for Chronic Diseases: What You Need to Know

While some chronic conditions result from your genetics, other conditions are determined by various factors. Several risk factors could increase your chances of developing certain chronic conditions. These risk factors can be divided into three categories. Let's consider each category and which factors put you at greater risk for chronic conditions.

Background Risk Factors

Background risk factors refer to things you have no control over or cannot change. They include factors like age, gender, and race. They also include factors like your heritage, as some ethnic groups are more prone to certain chronic conditions than others. While you cannot control these factors, it is important that you are aware of which chronic conditions you are more at risk for because of your background. For example, one study published in the *National Library of Medicine* found that "Patients from ethnic minorities with an acute stroke had 2- to fourfold greater likelihoods of stroke-related adverse outcomes and death than their Caucasian counterparts" (Fluck et al., 2023). Understanding your background-based risk can help you determine which tests you need (if any) to see if you have any of these conditions and how to prevent them from occurring or reduce your chances of developing them.

Behavioral Risk Factors

Certain behaviors or lifestyle habits also increase your risk of developing chronic conditions. If you pair these lifestyle habits with background risk factors, you will likely develop chronic conditions. However, these behavioral risk factors are known to cause chronic conditions even if you have no other risk factors. Behavioral risk factors include tobacco use and vaping, an unhealthy diet of highly processed or sugary foods, and an inactive lifestyle. A lack of sleep is also a behavioral risk factor that may lead to a compromised immune system, leading to chronic diseases.

Intermediate Risk Factors

Certain intermediate risk factors also increase your risk for some chronic diseases. Background risk factors or lifestyle risk factors often cause these risk factors. For example, an unhealthy diet may lead to increased blood pressure which could cause a stroke or heart disease. It might also cause you to become overweight and increase your blood glucose levels, which can lead to diabetes. Intermediate risk factors are the factors that result from one of the other risk factors and may lead to additional health conditions. It also makes managing a pre-existing chronic condition more challenging.

The Role of Genetics in Chronic Diseases: Myths and Realities

When you think of chronic disease, many thoughts may come to mind. And while some of these thoughts are backed by science, others are based on myths you may have heard before. Not all myths about chronic conditions are untrue. However, it is worth knowing which information you should take to heart, and which you should take with a pinch of salt. Here are some of the most common myths about chronic conditions and the realities these myths are based on.

Myth #1: Chronic Conditions are Caused by Genetics Alone

Many people think that genetics are the only cause of chronic diseases, or that they are a major contributor. However, that is not the case. One study published in the *National Library of Medicine* (Rappaport, 2016) found that genetics play a minor role in chronic conditions. You may therefore be at a slightly greater risk for developing certain chronic conditions based on your genetics, but this is not always the case. And, even if you are at a greater risk for developing a chronic condition based on your genetics, it does not mean that you cannot prevent or overcome these conditions.

Myth #2: There is Nothing You Can Do About Chronic Conditions Caused by Genetics

While many believe that you are doomed from the start if you are genetically at risk for certain chronic conditions, you can significantly reduce your chances of chronic conditions with lifestyle changes, regardless of your genetics. For example, if you have an increased risk of high blood pressure based on your genetics, it doesn't necessarily mean you will develop high blood pressure. You can reduce your chances of developing high blood pressure by leading an active lifestyle, eating a healthy, blood-pressure-regulating diet, and regularly having your blood pressure tested to get ahead of the disease.

Myth #3: A Healthy Lifestyle Negates the Risk of Chronic Conditions

Unfortunately, while lifestyle changes can help prevent and manage certain chronic conditions, even if you have a genetic risk for them, they cannot prevent all chronic conditions. Lifestyle changes make other chronic health conditions, including certain types of cancer, difficult to avoid. Furthermore, if you want to determine your risk for certain chronic conditions based on your genetics, you must have access to the right information and tests. If your family has some undiagnosed chronic conditions, it will be harder to determine your risk for developing it.

Understanding the common signs of a chronic condition can also help you determine if your family has chronic conditions. Furthermore, if there are, it is worth determining at which age your family members started showing signs of the chronic condition so you know when and what to be on the lookout for. While it is commonly believed that you have no control over your fate if you have a genetic risk for chronic disease, that is not the case. Knowledge is power; if you know the risk factors of a specific chronic disease, you can avoid getting it and manage it much sooner.

So while genetics does play a role in your risk for developing certain chronic conditions, it isn't necessarily the primary determiner. There are many myths and false information about chronic conditions and genetics. It is best to discuss your true risk of developing a chronic condition based on your genetics with your doctor to distinguish fact from fiction and help you base your treatment and prevention plan on your doctor's advice.

If you want to know more about your genetic risk for developing a chronic condition, you should consider genetic testing. Various other tests also diagnose chronic diseases and prevent them from developing and progressing.

Diagnosing Chronic Disease: Key Tests and Screening Processes

Chronic diseases are not always easy to detect at home. For example, you may feel tired and weak and think you have a vitamin deficiency when you have a tumor or other chronic condition. Therefore, it's important to go for regular health checkups to monitor your health and determine your risk for developing chronic conditions. Doctors may run a few key tests to rule out the presence of a chronic condition. Before running any tests, your doctor may take a full family history, where they will ask you if you know of any chronic conditions in your family. This can help them determine if you are at greater risk for developing one.

Furthermore, your doctor will ask you several questions, such as whether you smoke, your diet, and how active you are, to determine if your lifestyle puts you at greater risk for chronic conditions. If they deem it necessary, your doctor may order some tests to determine if you have a chronic disease. These tests may include:

Physical Examination

A physical exam can help determine your overall health and give a doctor an indication of whether you suffer from a chronic disease. Physical exams may include measuring your weight, heart rate, breathing, and overall condition.

Blood Tests

Blood tests can identify many health conditions, including certain chronic conditions. Increased blood glucose levels, cancer cells, thyroid problems, and signs of kidney, liver, and heart disease may be detected with a blood test. Doctors may run several blood tests to test for different chronic conditions.

Mammograms and Pap Smears

Mammograms and pap smears can help detect breast, ovarian, or cervical cancers, such as endometriosis, and other chronic conditions related to the female reproductive organs. Most women are recommended to see a gynecologist early to complete these tests and rule out any chronic conditions.

Colonoscopies

A colonoscopy helps rule out colon cancer or other chronic conditions related to the colon and intestines.

Colonoscopies are often done on patients who present with risk factors that may indicate colon cancer. A colonoscopy involves a tube with a camera placed inside the colon through the rectum to detect any physical problems, such as tumors.

Prostate Exams

Prostate exams are performed on men to determine their risk of prostate cancer. Prostate cancer is one of the leading cancers in men. A prostate exam is recommended yearly to determine your risk of prostate cancer and treat it if it arises. Fortunately, prostate cancer is highly treatable if detected early.

MRI and Other Imagery Tests

Suppose your blood test, physical exam, or medical history indicates a problem. In that case, your doctor may order an MRI or another imagery test to help them determine whether there is a bigger problem. Imagery tests can help doctors get a picture of your heart and other organs, which may show them if some tumors or deformities could point to a chronic condition.

Treating Chronic Diseases: A Holistic Approach

When you have been diagnosed with a chronic disease, there are several ways of going forward. There are many conventional medical treatments available for chronic conditions. However, a more holistic approach is also worth considering for healing certain chronic conditions, as it may have several additional health benefits. Furthermore, incorporating some holistic practices in addition to your medical treatments may provide an even better treatment plan for combating your chronic disease. As you may suspect based on the title of this book, fasting is one holistic approach you can include in your chronic disease prevention arsenal.

Dr. Otto Buchinger, founder of the Buchinger Wilhelmi Fasting Clinic, regarded fasting under experienced medical supervision and in an inspiring atmosphere not simply as a one-time corrective measure for an imbalanced state of health. He considered it to be the "true path of holistic medicine" and that it can help people to reach a more manageable lifestyle and lead them to the source of their self-healing powers (*History of the Company*, n.d.). This book will focus on fasting for chronic disease in much greater detail, so let's consider some other treatment plans available for chronic diseases.

Medications for Chronic Diseases: Benefits and Side Effects

Medications are a form of clinical treatment for chronic diseases. They are effective and based on scientific research. However, many medications have side effects, and you might have to use these medications lifelong to manage the symptoms of your disease. They are also expensive and are not always accessible through national health services or covered by health insurance.

Alternative Therapies for Chronic Diseases: What Works and What Doesn't

Of course, there are also many alternative therapies for chronic diseases. These include dietary and lifestyle changes, herbal medicine, and alternative treatments such as meditation and acupuncture. While some of these therapies effectively treat chronic diseases, not all are. They might also pose additional health risks. Some treatments, such as herbal medicine, might also interfere with your clinical treatment. Let's consider a few of these treatments in more detail and how they might help you overcome or manage your chronic disease.

Dietary Changes for Chronic Disease

Diet plays a massive role in your overall health and well-being. Certain dietary choices, such as a diet consisting of highly processed foods and sugars, may cause chronic conditions. Following a wholefoods diet that consists of plenty of high-quality proteins, fruits, vegetables, and healthy fats will boost your immune system and help prevent and manage chronic conditions. A ketogenic diet may also prove effective in treating certain chronic conditions (we will discuss this in greater detail in another chapter).

Exercise for Chronic Disease

There are many health benefits of exercise, and chronic disease prevention is one of them. Aiming for 150 minutes of exercise weekly can reduce your chances of developing chronic diseases like heart disease, diabetes, or stroke. Exercise also reduces stress and improves your bone density, helping to prevent osteoporosis. Combining cardiovascular, strength, and relaxation exercises can ensure you are getting well-rounded training and will deliver the most health benefits.

Meditation for Chronic Disease

Meditation is another holistic technique you can use to prevent and manage chronic disease. Meditation can help reduce the effects of oxidative stress on your body, improve sleep, and increase your mood. These factors can improve your natural immunity and make your body more resistant to chronic disease. Many chronic conditions are affected by stress, so stress relief should be one of your priorities when preventing and managing chronic disease.

Healthy Living for Chronic Disease

Other lifestyle changes, such as switching to a plastic-free lifestyle, avoiding the use of non-stick cookware, and avoiding products made of materials with carcinogenic effects are some other ways to prevent and manage chronic disease, especially certain types of cancer. While these techniques might not always be practical or affordable, every change you make will be beneficial to your health.

Coping with Chronic Disease: Strategies for Emotional and Mental Well-Being

Being diagnosed with a chronic condition may lead to emotional distress, depression, or anxiety. Therefore, it is crucial that you practice some techniques to improve your mental and emotional health. Therapy and self-care practices like journaling, meditation, and exercise can improve your mental health and help you cope with the emotional turmoil you may experience at this time.

Key Takeaway From Chapter 2

Chronic conditions are complex diseases with a longer incubation period and slow progress. Common chronic conditions include cancer and tumors, heart disease, diabetes, and kidney disease, to name a few. Certain risk factors, such as genetics, gender, race, and lifestyle choices, may increase your risk of developing chronic conditions. Fortunately, with regular health checkups, you can detect a chronic disease much sooner and work on getting it treated. Many treatments are available for chronic conditions, each with advantages and disadvantages.

Chapter 3:

Understanding Fasting

This is the third book in my series about the wonderful advantages of fasting. The first two books, *Gut Health and Fasting for Beginners* and *Revitalize Your Brain After 40 With Fasting* explained fasting models in much greater detail, which is why I strongly recommend you read them (they are available on Amazon). For those who have not read these books, this chapter will focus on a condensed version of fasting, the different types of fasting models, and how they work. This will give you a great idea of what you are getting into when you start a fasting regime.

Different Fasting Models

Fasting is a type of restrictive eating. While many consider it a diet, it is not so much a diet as an eating "schedule." Instead of determining what you can eat, fasting limits when you can. By only allowing food intake at certain times and for certain periods, you will automatically consume fewer calories, assisting in weight loss and weight management. As such, many people use fasting as a weight loss method. But there are many other health benefits of fasting, including reducing the symptoms of chronic diseases. We'll discuss various advantages of fasting later in this chapter. For now, though, let's consider the different fasting models and how each works.

Intermittent Fasting

Intermittent fasting is one of the best-known fasting models. It consists of periods of fasting which are interrupted by an eating period. There are different kinds of intermittent fasting models, including

- **Alternate Day Fasting:** This fasting model involves having higher-calorie days when you eat your normal foods and low-calorie days when you eat far less food than you normally do. As the name suggests, you alternate between these high-calorie and low-calorie days.

- **5/2 Fasting:** This is an example of alternate-day fasting. However, instead of alternating day-for-day between higher and lower calories, you would choose two days in that week during which you eat nothing to only a few calories. You would eat as you normally do for the rest of the week.

- **Extended Fasting:** With extended fasting, you would choose a time during the week for which you fast for a much longer period, such as 24, 36, or 48 hours. Extended fasting is also known as prolonged fasting (which we will discuss in more detail in the following chapter). In some cases, extended fasting may also endure for several days, or even weeks, depending on the chronic health condition you are combatting.

- **Time Restricted Eating:** This is one of the best-known fasting models. It involves having an eating window that disrupts your fasting period. People often incorporate time-restricted eating in the following increments: 12/12, 8/16, and 10/14. The times describe how long their eating window is during the day and how long their fasting window is.

Dry Fasting

As the name suggests, dry fasting is a fasting model where you cannot consume any liquids during your fasting window. You can combine dry fasting with intermittent fasting or other fasting models. However, you run the risk of dehydration with dry fasting, making it unsuitable for those with kidney problems or other chronic or acute health conditions.

Water Fasting

Water fasting is the opposite of dry fasting. You can also combine it with other fasting models. However, while dry fasting restricts fluid intake during the fasting window, water fasting allows for the intake of fluids during this time. This reduces the chance of dehydration, making you feel fuller during your fasting window since you can consume fluids.

Fast Mimicking

Fast mimicking is a fasting model that doesn't actually require any true fasting. Instead, you eat foods that are low enough in calories to trick your body into the ketogenic state (during which your body burns fat for energy instead of carbohydrates). Fast mimicking is also known as a Prolon fast. This fasting method allows you to eat certain foods from a selected list during your fasting window. While you can eat particular foods, you are restricted with what you can eat, and the foods on the Prolon diet tend to be expensive.

Fasting and Angiogenesis

One of the positive effects of fasting is angiogenesis. According to the *National Cancer Institute*, "Angiogenesis is the formation of new blood vessels. This process involves the migration, growth, and differentiation of endothelial cells, which line the inside wall of blood vessels" (*Angiogenesis Inhibitors*, 2018). Certain fasting models, including intermittent fasting, have a positive effect on angiogenesis, which has many positive health effects on the body. The first book in this series, *Gut Health and Fasting for Beginners*, has an extended section on fasting and Angiogenesis in Chapter 7, where we explained how angiogenesis works and how it can prevent certain types of cancers, regulate blood sugar levels, and improve your immune system, among other things. One study performed on ischemic rats found the following effects of intermittent fasting on angiogenesis (Liu et al., 2023)

- It increases microvessel density.

- It activates certain growth differentiator factor pathways (which play a role in the body's cellular regeneration system).

- It stimulates the proliferation of endothelial cells.

- It promotes regional cerebral blood flow.

- It regulates the total vessel surface area.

- It regulates the number of microvessel branch points.

Increased angiogenesis has a significant effect on your overall health. It can manage and prevent certain chronic conditions, including cancer, heart disease, stroke, and kidney disease. By increasing cell regeneration, angiogenesis helps your body recover faster. The strengthened blood vessels will be more resistant to decay, helping to prevent heart disease. Furthermore, by increasing blood flow to the brain, your cognitive abilities will remain intact, which can help your body combat chronic conditions naturally.

The fact that intermittent fasting is proven to increase angiogenesis already tells you some compelling reasons why you should consider fasting for preventing and managing chronic health conditions. And yet, angiogenesis is not the only health benefit associated with fasting. Fasting provides many other health benefits too. As discussed in the first two books of this series, fasting can significantly improve gut and brain health. Let us now consider the general health benefits of fasting before we do a deeper study of the impact of fasting on chronic diseases.

The Effects of Fasting on the Body

Before we delve into the effects of fasting on chronic diseases specifically, it is worth discovering how chronic diseases affect your body in general. This will give you a better idea of why many people follow a fasting lifestyle, even if they don't have a chronic condition. It will also give you a better idea of how fasting benefits chronic diseases. So, let's consider the effects of fasting on the body before we explore how these effects impact chronic conditions.

How Does Fasting Influence the Body?

Your body goes through many processes, most relying on the energy gained from the food you eat. And yet some significant health benefits result from the functions your body goes through when you don't eat. As you can imagine, fasting significantly influences your metabolism, which explains the health benefits of fasting on your gut. But what are some other effects of fasting on your body and health?

Fasting Leads to Lower Insulin Levels

When you eat, your body converts the carbs and sugars into glucose which feeds your body and cells. Your body also releases a hormone called insulin to manage blood glucose levels. The problem is that too much insulin in the blood can lead to hormonal imbalances. When you fast, your body has more time to break down the available glucose and use it for energy. Then, it supplements that energy with stored fat that does not require insulin management. As such, fasting reduces the insulin levels in your blood, which can help prevent and manage certain chronic conditions.

Fasting Leaves More Time for Cellular Repair and Regeneration

Autophagy is the body's cellular regeneration system. When you fast, your body has more time for autophagy, which involves breaking down damaged cells and reusing them to repair and make new ones. Since cellular damage often results in certain chronic conditions, fasting can help to improve cellular regeneration and help prevent and manage cellular aging, which leads to increased overall health. Increased cellular repair may also combat certain chronic conditions, especially those more prevalent with aging.

Fasting Increases HGH Levels

Human growth hormone, or HGH, is responsible for many bodily functions. HGH is not only responsible for muscle growth and tissue repair, but it also helps your body burn fat. Unfortunately, your HGH levels decrease dramatically after the age of 30. HGH is released at the 13th hour when fasting and increases by 500% when one reaches the 48-hour mark (Berg, 2018). Increased HGH levels may also prevent chronic diseases and improve overall health and well-being.

Fasting Helps With Hormone Regulation

Did you know that there are more than 50 different kinds of hormones in the human body? These hormones are regulated by the endocrine system, which includes parts of the brain, reproductive organs, thyroid, and more. Your hormones are affected by many internal and external factors, including insulin levels and gut health. Therefore, since fasting improves gut health and reduces insulin levels in the blood, it also helps with hormone regulation. This has a significant effect on your overall health. It can also help prevent and manage chronic conditions connected to hormone fluctuations.

How do These Factors Affect Chronic Conditions?

Now that we have discussed some basic effects of fasting on the body (there are many more that can be discussed in detail when you want to discover the effects of fasting on certain body parts, including the gut and the brain), we can consider how these factors affect chronic diseases. While all the above-mentioned factors affect your health in general, they also have some specific health benefits relating to chronic conditions. How can you use fasting to improve chronic conditions?

Fasting Reduces Inflammation

One of the positive health effects of fasting is that it reduces inflammation. According to *Harvard Medical School*, chronic inflammation is associated with several chronic conditions, including cancer, arthritis, heart disease, diabetes, and bowel diseases like Chrons and ulcerative colitis (*Understanding Acute and Chronic Inflammation*, 2020). Fasting is shown to reduce inflammation throughout your body. Furthermore, fasting also reduces oxidative stress, which can also lead to several chronic conditions.

Fasting Leads to Cell Reparation

Fasting can also lead to cell reparation. As explained above, fasting increases autophagy, which helps repair damaged or dead cells faster. Cellular repair can help keep your organs, tissue, and blood vessels functioning optimally. This can help your body combat several chronic conditions. Furthermore, if your body is stronger, it can manage chronic conditions better, increasing your quality of life despite having a chronic condition.

Fasting Can Help Manage Your Weight

Fasting puts your body in ketosis, which means that your body starts burning fat for energy instead of sugars. When your body runs out of readily available fat, it will start burning stored fat or energy. This will help you burn fat and reduce your chances of becoming obese or suffering from obese-related chronic conditions, such as diabetes and strokes, to name a few.

Fasting Improves Metabolism

Fasting also assists with your metabolism, which might help decrease your chances of certain chronic conditions. For example, if your metabolism is slower, your nutrient absorption will also be compromised. In addition, certain chronic conditions, such as chronic constipation and colon cancer, are related to a compromised metabolism (Scheurlen et al., 2020). A slower metabolism could also lead to weight gain, obesity, and chronic health conditions related to obesity. Therefore, since fasting improves your metabolism and nutrient absorption, it can reduce your risk of developing certain chronic diseases.

Key Takeaway From Chapter 3

Many different fasting models can help reduce chronic conditions. Some of the most common fasting methods include intermittent fasting, water fasting, dry fasting, and fast mimicking. Fasting leads to angiogenesis, which is the process during which your endothelial cells are repaired, your vein and artery walls are strengthened, and your cerebral blood flow is increased. Fasting also leads to lower insulin levels, increased cellular repair, increased HGH levels, and hormone regulation. As a result, fasting reduces inflammation, assists with cellular reparation, assists with weight management, and improves your metabolism. These factors all have a positive effect on your body and may help to reduce chronic conditions.

Chapter 4:

The Prolonged Fasting

Regimen

While you could gain health benefits and see improvement in chronic conditions with any fasting regime, some evidence suggests that a prolonged fast (PF) significantly improves chronic diseases. Prolonged fasting also has many other health benefits, which we will discuss in this chapter. But there are also some precautions when fasting for an extended period; not everyone is suitable for prolonged fasting. Therefore, we will discuss prolonged fasting in detail in the following three chapters.

In this chapter, you will learn what prolonged fasting is, the benefits of prolonged fasting, prolonged fasting mistakes, and who should not consider prolonged fasting. If you are considering a more direct fasting approach to target your chronic conditions, then prolonged fasting might be the way to go.

What is Prolonged Fasting?

While there is no standardized definition of prolonged fasting, the term generally relates to a fasting period of 36 hours or more. There is no predetermined period for how long you should fast during a prolonged fast, and the period you choose to do a prolonged fast will depend on many factors, including previous fasting experience, tolerance, overall health, and age. Prolonged fasting typically allows for certain no-calorie beverages, including water, tea (without milk or sugar), and electrolyte drinks. Due to the extended period of this fast, prolonged fasting should not be combined with dry fasting, as it could lead to dehydration.

Prolonged Fasting (PF) vs. Intermittent Fasting (IF)

Intermittent fasting is one of the most popular fasting models. As the name suggests, it involves intermittent periods of fasting and eating (eat-stop-eat). So how does this differ from a prolonged fast? According to Laura Bais (2023) from *Boxrox*, "While intermittent fasting means interval eating, i.e., you eat in an eight-hour window and fast the other 16 hours, prolonged fasting means not eating for at least 36 hours." Both intermittent fasting and prolonged fasting can yield impressive results for weight loss and improved health.

The primary difference between these fasting models is that intermittent fasting has a fasting and eating period within a 24-hour window. In contrast, prolonged fasting typically occurs over the span of a week or month, depending on the duration of the fast and your goals.

Why Prolonged Fasting?

Considering there are so many fasting models, and most of them are not quite as intense or demanding as prolonged fasting, you may wonder why prolonged fasting is the most beneficial for chronic conditions (this is, after all, the purpose of this book). The reality is that the longer you fast the more metabolic switches you pull in your body, and the more healing occurs. Prolonged fasting has many amazing benefits, which we will discuss in the following section. The general idea is that prolonged fasting resets your body to some extent. All the benefits we have discussed in the previous chapter and in books 1 and 2 of this series, increase during a prolonged fast, as your body has more time for autophagy, cellular regeneration, hormonal balancing, and more.

Prolonged fasting has also been shown to help manage autoimmune diseases, balance testosterone levels, remove aging cells that could cause cancer if they multiply, and increase telomere length (Pelz, 2023). This means prolonged fasting may yield results faster than other fasting models, and you can see positive effects much sooner.

A Word of Caution About Prolonged Fast

Before we delve into the various benefits of prolonged fasting, I would like to caution you about this fasting model. Prolonged/long-term fasting is healthy, but it does come with risks if done incorrectly. You shouldn't do a prolonged fast for too long (over 7 days), and it's not worth attempting until you master regular fasting daily for at least several months. Your body needs some time to adjust to any fasting model, and jumping into prolonged fasting without preparing your body could lead to unpleasant side effects. Prolonged fasting can be done safely but should always be done under the close supervision of a medical professional.

Benefits of Prolonged Fasting

Now that we have the word of caution out of the way and you understand what prolonged fasting is let's consider the benefits of prolonged fasting. These benefits relate not only to chronic conditions but also to general health and well-being. So, let's consider the health benefits of prolonged fasting and why you should consider this fasting model if you wish to improve your health.

Getting Rid of Societal Food Addiction

One of the reasons why we don't typically fast anymore is because there is no need to. Most of us are privileged enough that we have a fridge or freezer to store food in for longer periods. We also have access to shops year-round, meaning that we never experience food shortages, which would lead to fasting. However, people have become so accustomed to eating on any occasion, where food should be a source of energy for survival, it has become a show of wealth, and many companies and franchises create a sense of food addiction by associating food with success, likeability, and experiences. As RJ so appropriately said in *Over The Hedge*, "We (animals) eat to live. These guys (humans) live to eat!" (*Over the Hedge*, 2006).

Prolonged fasting can adjust your perspective of food, helping you break the tradition of societal food addiction. Instead of relying on food to help you socialize, you will use other methods and activities to socialize with loved ones. You will also learn to appreciate food and food availability more.

Leading to More Metabolic Flexibility

You may have heard that having a set eating schedule is good. Breakfast, lunch, and dinner; that's what we all were taught. However, considering how our ancestors lived, you will realize that having a set time to eat three meals a day is not natural for the human body. In fact, the human body is designed to go days without food, which is why your body stores fat as a reserve to use during this time. Prolonged fasting leads to metabolic flexibility. Your body will relearn to switch between burning carbs and fat for fuel, assisting in weight management and helping you to function optimally even while fasting. This means you will no longer feel dizzy or faint after skipping breakfast.

Preventing Major Health Conditions

Of course, prolonged fasting can also help prevent major health conditions. According to the *University of Southern California*, each time you fast for a prolonged period, the reduction in white blood cells increases the rate of stem cell regeneration of new immune cells (Wu, 2014). This allows your body to fight illnesses more effectively, which can help prevent chronic and acute conditions. A six-month study looking at mice and humans undergoing chemotherapy treatment found that fasting for 72 hours resulted in significant health improvements due to blood cells and other toxins being cleared from the body (Longo & Mattson, 2014). This study by Longo and Mattson (2014) also found the following:

> "In rodents, intermittent or periodic fasting protects against diabetes, cancers, heart disease, and neurodegeneration, while in humans, it helps reduce obesity, hypertension, asthma, and rheumatoid arthritis. Thus, fasting can potentially delay aging and help prevent and treat diseases while minimizing the side effects caused by chronic dietary interventions."

As you can see, prolonged fasting has many impressive health benefits. Its health benefits are not only relevant to those combating chronic conditions but to preventing and reducing the symptoms of many other conditions too. As you can see from the study by Longo and Mattson (2014), prolonged fasting also has some benefits for those already suffering from a chronic condition, such as cancer. Therefore, it is never too late to try prolonged fasting and consider how it may improve your health.

How Long Should You Fast?

The longest recorded fast lasted for 382 days (Bais, 2023). During this period, the patient was closely monitored by various healthcare professionals. He was also obese when the experiment started, so he had sufficient energy deposits for his body to use while fasting. He lost a total of 276 pounds. But this was an extreme case performed in the name of science. Most people choose between 36 and 72-hour fasts. Some people fast for even longer than that. And while you can safely fast for up to seven days, it is not recommended to do so for longer than that without medical supervision and a clean bill of health before starting the fast.

Regardless of how long you choose to do a prolonged fast, you must drink enough fluids, including electrolytes, while doing a prolonged fast. How long you do a prolonged fast will depend on your fasting experience, goals, and underlying health conditions before starting a fast in the first place.

How Does the Body Survive Prolonged Fasting?

As you may have grown up with the idea that you must eat frequent meals to stay healthy, you may wonder how the body survives prolonged fasting. There are three stages of prolonged fasting, during which the body makes several changes to accommodate the lack of new carbohydrate sources. Let's consider the different fasting stages and how your body survives prolonged fasting.

Fed State

This is the first state of fasting and occurs immediately after you eat (until about three hours later). During this time, your body digests the food you have eaten. Many hormones are involved in this process, including ghrelin, leptin, and insulin. Since you have just eaten, your body doesn't experience major changes in the fed state.

Early Fasting State

The early fasting state lasts between 3-4 and 18 hours after your last meal. This is when you will start seeing an increase in certain activities that help your body survive during this state. Your body starts secreting glucagon, which stabilizes your blood sugar levels. Furthermore, your body starts using glycogen for energy. The hormones involved in this fasting stage include glucagon, cortisol, epinephrine, and HGH.

Fasting State

After the 18-hour mark, you will enter the fasting state. This state lasts between 18 and 48 hours. By this time, your body will start burning fat for fuel as it has entered the ketogenic state. Furthermore, your body may also enter autophagy during the fasting state. The fasting state is where you can experience the most weight loss benefits, as ketosis burns stored fat for energy.

Prolonged Fasting State

Finally, after 48 hours, you will enter the prolonged fasting state. This state will lead to your insulin levels dropping further and your ketones increasing further. The breakdown of amino acids also decreases to preserve muscle mass. Overall, the more body fat you have, the longer your body can survive in the fasting state. However, that doesn't mean you should fast indefinitely. In fact, some people should not try prolonged fasting at all.

Who Must Not Embrace Prolonged Fasting

While prolonged fasting offers some impressive health benefits, it is not a solution for everyone. In some situations, fasting might not be a suitable healthcare option. The following factors might make it unsuitable for you to attempt prolonged fasting.

Pregnancy

If you are pregnant, your body requires more energy and nutrients. Furthermore, your body won't handle the stress of prolonged (or any) fasting when you are pregnant, as it is already under more stress because of the pregnancy. Therefore, prolonged fasting is not a viable option if you are pregnant, regardless of which health conditions you may wish to combat.

Breastfeeding Mothers

Just like when you are pregnant, your body requires more nutrients when breastfeeding. It takes a lot of energy to produce the milk your body needs, and some of the necessary hormones may be affected by the lack of energy during a fast. Unfortunately, this means you cannot start a prolonged fast if you are breastfeeding.

People With Eating Disorders

If you have an eating disorder, you must be mindful of fasting. Despite being healthy in many ways, prolonged fasting can transform into another way to feed your disorder as a form of abuse. Therefore, only consider prolonged fasting if you have recovered from your eating disorder and if you have gotten the all-clear from your doctor and specialist. Even if you have recovered from your earring disorder, prolonged fasting may trigger it, so you should think twice before embracing this fasting regimen.

People Taking Certain Medications

While fasting can help reduce many chronic conditions, it might not always be a suitable solution. If you take medications that require you to eat regularly, prolonged fasting may do more harm than good. In this case, only consider prolonged fasting if you have consulted your doctor first.

Prolonged Fasting Mistakes

We'll discuss the proper way to break a fast in the following chapter. However, some common fasting mistakes are worth mentioning now so you get an idea of what you should not do when you try prolonged fasting. These mistakes can sometimes cause health problems. In most cases, though, they will make your fasting experience much worse than it would have been had you followed the right protocols. Some prolonged fasting mistakes to avoid, according to prolonged fasting expert Dr. Eric Berg (2022), include

- Breaking your fast with carbohydrates.

- Intensely exercising while on a prolonged fast.

- Overeating when you break your fast.

- Consuming protein powders when breaking a fast.

These mistakes will make you feel ill when breaking the prolonged fast, which might make you hesitant to try it again. So, you can make things much easier for yourself when breaking the fast if you avoid these mistakes and follow the tips for effectively undertaking and breaking a prolonged fast. Speaking of which, how do you start a prolonged fast safely?

Undertaking a Prolonged Fast Safely

When undertaking a prolonged fast, it's crucial that you do so safely. Many factors may affect your suitability for prolonged fasting, as explained in the previous section. However, if you want to safely engage in a prolonged fast, there are a few things to remember. The first thing is to consult your doctor or healthcare practitioner about the safety of prolonged fasting in your specific case.

Another safety measure is to drink plenty of fluids and electrolytes during the fast so you don't become dehydrated.

Furthermore, monitoring your well-being (how you feel, your weight and measurements, and possibly your ketones) can help determine if everything is okay while fasting. Finally, breaking the fast correctly is just as important as undertaking it correctly. Not concluding a fast in the right way could undo all your hard work, meaning you endured a prolonged fast for nothing.

Hacks to Make Prolonged Fast Effortless

As we have mentioned before, practicing intermittent fasting and following a ketogenic diet before embarking on a prolonged fast makes things easier, and it is strongly recommended that you become acquainted with intermittent fasting or other fasting models before undertaking a prolonged fast. But no matter how much experience you have with other fasting models, it will be a challenge if it's your first time trying a prolonged fast. Fortunately, there are some things you can try to make your first prolonged fasting experience much easier, including the following:

- Drink enough water and electrolytes to keep your body hydrated and prevent mineral and sodium loss.

- Consider a vitamin B supplement (vitamin B is typically found in red meat and healthy fats) to assist with normal bodily functions and improve ketosis.

- Consider taking EDTA to assist with detoxification.

EDTA is a chelating agent that binds to metals in the body. Metals such as arsenic, mercury, iron, aluminum, and lead are all found in your body. These metals have some negative health effects, and your body could benefit from reducing them. One way to reduce these metals and increase detoxification is by taking supplemental EDTA. While you wouldn't need to take EDTA when you are not fasting, as it occurs in dark green vegetables (*What are the Health Benefits*, 2015), you might benefit from taking EDTA supplements when prolonged fasting.

Take care when using EDTA, however, as it absorbs beneficial and harmful minerals. This is why a mineral supplement and electrolytes will be a great addition during a prolonged fast (Berg, 2018).

When to Break a Prolonged Fast

When you first start a prolonged fast, you may have a predetermined hour at which you plan to break the fast. That is beneficial as it will give you something to focus on. However, there is also a solid argument to make for letting your body decide for you. Your body will tell you when it is ready to eat again. As you become more accustomed to prolonged fasting, you will learn to listen to your body more closely and you will intuitively know when it is time to break the fast. When you complete your first prolonged fast, you may not be as attuned to your body yet, and you may think that it needs food the first time you feel hungry. Just hang in there; you will eventually get the hang of things and learn to trust your body more.

Key Takeaway From Chapter 4

Prolonged fasting has some impressive health benefits relating to chronic conditions. Prolonged fasting is a fasting model that requires fasting for more than 36 hours. It is often compared with intermittent fasting. While both models alternate between eat-fast-eat, intermittent fasting typically runs on a 24-hour loop, while prolonged fasting runs on a much longer loop, such as a week or month. While prolonged fasting has many health benefits, it is not suitable for everyone, including pregnant women and those with a history of eating disorders. You can make prolonged fasting much easier on yourself if you follow the right protocols, like drinking enough fluids and eating the right foods when you break the fast.

Chapter 5:

Breaking a Prolonged Fast

Now that you understand how prolonged fasting works and some of its benefits, it's time to take a deeper dive into how you can properly break a prolonged fast. As mentioned in the previous chapter, correctly concluding a prolonged fast is just as important as fasting. If you don't break your fast the right way, you may experience some unpleasant side effects. Therefore, this chapter will help you understand how to correctly break a prolonged fast to get the most health benefits. We'll discuss fast-breaking mistakes in more detail, what refeeding syndrome is and why you should avoid it, and how to make the perfect fast-breaking soup to ease your body into tolerating food again.

Fast Breaking is as Important as Fasting

When you have endured your first prolonged fast, you are probably very excited to start eating again, especially if there are foods you have been craving during the fasting period. However, if you don't break a prolonged fast correctly, you may shock your body, which could lead to several unpleasant side effects, including:

- bloating

- gas

- nausea and vomiting

- diarrhea

- passing undigested foods

After experiencing some of these side effects, you may be more hesitant to try a prolonged fast again. Furthermore, if you eat the wrong kinds of food when you first break a prolonged fast, your blood sugar levels may spike, which could cause other health problems. Therefore, concluding a prolonged fast correctly is just as important as following the correct fasting protocols.

While there aren't as many strict protocols when undertaking a shorter fast, you must remember that your body has been without food for some time during a prolonged fast. It has made several adaptations to survive without food, as discussed in Chapter 3 of this book and books 1 and 2 of this series.

But why do some people experience these side effects when breaking a prolonged fast? The reason is that when you enter a prolonged fasting state, your body stops producing as many digestive enzymes. It no longer needs them, as there isn't new food entering the body that needs digesting (Ramos, n.d.). When you break the fast, your body won't have the digestive enzymes available for digesting the food you consume.

This means that if you consume foods that are difficult to digest (such as heavy proteins or complex carbohydrates), your body will have difficulty digesting those foods, which could lead to digestive distress. So, before we discuss the best practices for concluding a fast correctly, let's consider the most common fast-breaking mistakes.

Fast-Breaking Mistakes

While we listed the most common fast-breaking mistakes in the previous chapter, it didn't really explain why you should avoid these mistakes and why they are mistakes in the first place. Allow me to elaborate on the common fast-breaking mistakes and why you should avoid them. According to Dr. Eric Berg (2022), a seasoned professional in the world of prolonged fasting, these are the five most common fasting mistakes and why you should avoid them.

Concluding Your Fast With Carbohydrates and Sugars

During a prolonged fast, your body produces more stem cells (Berg, 2022). These stem cells are ready to go where your body needs them and repair other cells in your body. But when you consume too many carbohydrates and sugars (including fruits) when breaking a fast, those stem cells will convert into fat cells, as your body will suspect it needs more fat cells to store excess energy from these foods. Therefore, consuming carbohydrates and sugars when concluding a fast can undo all your body's progress during the prolonged fasting period.

Engaging in Intense Exercise During and Immediately After Prolonged Fasting

You may have read that it is perfectly safe (and beneficial) to continue with an intense exercise routine while fasting. This is absolutely true when intermittent fasting. However, when you are doing a prolonged fast, your body is placed under a lot of stress. It is focused on recovery and preservation. Engaging in intense exercise at this time can do more harm than good. It can place even more stress on your body. Your body might also not have enough electrolytes to support your heart and organs during exercise at this time. Instead of starting training immediately after a prolonged fast, allow your body to replenish its reserves and feel rejuvenated before continuing your training routine.

Overeating When You Break a Prolonged Fast

As discussed in the previous section, your digestive system goes to sleep when fasting. This means it will not be ready to process large quantities of food simultaneously. As such, you must start with small meals to wake your digestive system up and give it time to produce the enzymes and acids needed for proper digestion. If you overeat when concluding a prolonged fast, you may experience some of the side effects mentioned above.

Taking Apple Cider Vinegar During or After a Prolonged Fast

Apple cider vinegar (ACV) is said to aid with your digestive system. This is why some people take ACV during a fast to help "awaken" the digestive system and reduce the symptoms of digestive distress when breaking a fast. However, your body enters ketosis when you are doing a prolonged fast. According to Dr. Berg (2022), ketones are acidic. This means your body will already be quite acidic during a prolonged fast. Drinking apple cider vinegar after a fast will only cause your body to become more acidic, leading to several health conditions and physical discomfort.

Consuming Protein Powder When Concluding a Prolonged Fast

Something like a protein powder is an excellent way of breaking a prolonged fast, as it is fast to consume, high in protein, and has less volume than eating solid food. However, protein powders are some of the foods that increase your insulin levels the most. They are also extremely low in fat, compromising the body's ketosis. Therefore, instead of opting for a protein powder, consume an egg or whole protein (with fat) instead.

Refeeding Syndrome

While refeeding syndrome is a fairly common problem that is surprisingly poorly studied. Refeeding syndrome not only occurs in persons breaking a prolonged fast but may occur in other circumstances, such as people recovering from an eating disorder. As you will see in this section, the refeeding syndrome has some unpleasant, potentially dangerous, or even fatal side effects. Therefore, it is crucial that you follow the correct protocols when concluding an extended fast to avoid accidentally triggering refeeding syndrome and undoing all the positive effects the fast has on your body.

What is Refeeding Syndrome?

A study published in the *National Library of Medicine* describes refeeding syndrome as "The potentially fatal shifts in fluids and electrolytes that may occur in malnourished patients receiving artificial refeeding. These shifts result from hormonal and metabolic changes and may cause serious clinical complications" (Mehanna et al., 2008). While refeeding syndrome is quite common, it is not often discussed. Furthermore, refeeding syndrome is often overlooked as a potential danger when breaking a fast or recovering from an eating disorder.

While you may think that your body will need a lot of food immediately when you break a prolonged fast, and while you will likely be hungry enough to devour a table of food, that is certainly not the best course of action to take when you break a fast. You may also wonder if, apart from experiencing digestive distress, there are any other dangers of refeeding syndrome. And if so, what are they?

Dangers of Refeeding After Prolonged Fast

There are quite a few unpleasant and potentially life-threatening dangers of refeeding syndrome. As you can imagine, your body undergoes great stress during a prolonged fast. So many processes occur in the body, from ketosis to autophagy, that your body will be sensitive to sudden changes, including reintroducing foods. As you already know, your digestive system also slows or goes dormant during a prolonged fast. So, if you introduce too much food at once after a prolonged fast, you will overwhelm your digestive system, which could lead to a host of problems. But more serious health conditions could also occur from refeeding syndrome, including depletion of the following minerals.

Phosphorus

Phosphate is a crucial intercellular mineral. It is responsible for many functions, including cellular structure and intercellular energy storage. If you experience refeeding syndrome, your cells will become depleted of phosphorus, which could cause many problems throughout the body and even threaten your heart health.

Magnesium

According to Mehanna et al. (2008), magnesium is another intercellular mineral responsible for many functions, including the structural integrity of RNA, DNA, and ribosomes. Depletion of magnesium could lead to neuromuscular complications and cardiac dysfunction.

Potassium

A potassium deficiency in the blood is known as hypokalemia. It occurs during refeeding syndrome and can lead to severe health conditions, including cardiac arrest or arrhythmias. Potassium is a crucial mineral for heart health.

Glucose

Instead of causing a glucose depletion, the refeeding syndrome may cause a spike of glucose in the bloodstream, which could lead to hyperglycemia and its sequelae of osmotic diuresis, dehydration, metabolic acidosis, and ketoacidosis" (Mehanna et al., 2008). Increased glucose levels may cause respiratory failure, fatty liver, and increased carbon dioxide production.

Vitamins

Vitamin deficiencies may occur at any time during a prolonged fast. However, a thiamine deficiency is more common during refeeding syndrome. Unfortunately, a thiamine deficiency can lead to various health conditions, including Wernicke's encephalopathy and Korsakoff's syndrome.

Fluids, Sodium, and Nitrogen

Refeeding syndrome may also lead to more frequent urination, which causes an increased depletion of nitrogen, sodium, and fluids, all crucial for optimal health. If these minerals and fluids are depleted, you are at greater risk for congestive heart failure, arrhythmias, and pulmonary edema.

You may wonder why all these things occur from overfeeding. The primary reason why this happens is because of the insulin spikes your body experiences when you first consume food after a prolonged fast. These insulin spikes lead to intercellular changes, where your cells absorb many minerals listed above. This leads to too few minerals being left in the blood, which is why you are at risk for heart problems and various other health conditions when experiencing refeeding syndrome. So, how can you avoid refeeding syndrome?

How to Avoid Refeeding Syndrome

Considering how serious refeeding syndrome is, you may wish to know how you can avoid suffering from it when concluding a prolonged fast. Fortunately, following the correct protocols is rather easy to avoid refeeding syndrome. This includes starting with small meals that consist of protein, fats, or fermented foods when you first break your prolonged fast. Dr. Eric Berg (2018) mentions foods like kimchi, a whole egg, half an avocado, or some broth. Then, wait a few hours for those foods to digest properly and your digestive system to wake up.

When you have waited a few hours after eating your first fast-breaking meal, you can eat another small meal, such as a small salad, perhaps a few carbs (like oats or sweet potatoes), or some more eggs. Continue eating small meals while giving your body the proper rest and nutrition it needs while you are recovering from the prolonged fast. Another crucial thing to do that will help prevent refeeding syndrome is to drink enough fluids and electrolytes to account for any mineral loss that might occur when concluding the prolonged fast.

The Perfect Soup for a Prolonged Fast

One of the best ways to break a prolonged fast is with soup. Soups are packed with vitamins and minerals, easy to digest, and don't involve much energy to consume. One of the chefs, Hubert Hohler, at B*uchinger Wilhelmi Clinic*, a leading clinic in the field of prolonged fasting, shared his recipe for the perfect prolonged fasting soup (Wilhelmi, 2021). He mentions that you only want to use between one and three kinds of vegetables when making this soup, as you don't want to overwhelm the digestive system. For example, you can use onion, a bit of potato for a creamier texture, and carrots for your prolonged fasting soup. Then, you can also choose three types of herbs to add to the soup, such as lemongrass, ginger, or bay leaves.

To make the soup, simply chop around 14 ounces of vegetables and sauté them in a pan (without any fat). Add the spices and four cups of water to the pot when the vegetables have wilted. Cook the vegetables until they are tender. Then, remove the hard herbs (lemongrass and bay leaves) before blending the soup. Pass the soup through a strainer to ensure it is thin enough to not activate your colon. Finally, add salt to taste, and then you are ready to enjoy your soup! This soup is intended to be enjoyed during a prolonged fast, as you will still be consuming some calories now.

However, if you are making a soup for breaking your fast, you can also add some bone broth to the soup for additional nutrients and taste. You could add vegetable broth to the soup for a more concentrated flavor. However, it's important to ensure that you use an organic vegetable broth that does not contain added salt or preservatives. Chef Hubert recommends eating one cup of this soup at a time. You could eat more than that, but it would depend on how you feel. This is the perfect soup to enjoy both during and after a prolonged fast, as it won't lead to refeeding syndrome, and it will make you feel satisfied, hydrated, and nourished.

Key Takeaway From Chapter 5

Concluding a prolonged fast is just as important as following the correct prolonged fasting protocols. If you don't break a prolonged fast correctly, you will be at greater risk of experiencing digestive distress (bloating, gas, nausea, and more). You will also be at greater risk for developing refeeding syndrome, which occurs due to insulin spikes and can be life-threatening. Therefore, it's important to break your fast correctly and avoid refeeding syndrome. You can eat small, simple meals when you break the fast, such as eggs, avocado, or bone broth. You can also make vegetable soup to enjoy during and after your fasting period.

Make a Difference With Your Review

Unlock the Power of Kindness

If you want others to be happy, practice compassion. If you want to be happy, practice compassion. –Dalai Lama

People who give without expecting anything in return live longer, happier lives. So, if we've got a shot at that while we're here together, I'm gonna try my best!

I have a question for you...

Would you help someone you've never met, even if you never got any credit for it?

Who is this person, you ask? They are like you. Or, at least, how you used to be. Maybe feeling tired and run down from a chronic condition, wanting to feel better, and needing help, but not sure where to turn.

My mission is to make ***Fasting Secrets for Chronic Conditions*** a book that can help everyone. Everything I do comes from that goal. And, the only way for ME to reach that goal is by reaching...well...everyone.

This is where you come in. Most people do judge a book by its cover (and its reviews!). So, here's my request on behalf of someone struggling with a chronic condition that you've never met:

Please help that person by leaving this book a review.

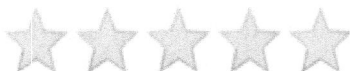

★ ★ ★ ★ ★

Your gift costs no money and takes less than a minute, but it can change someone's life forever. Your review could help...

- one more person experience relief from their symptoms.

- one more person step towards a life free from chronic pain and inflammation.

- one more person reclaim their energy and vitality.

- one more family enjoy more quality time together.

To get that warm, fuzzy feeling and help someone for real, all you have to do is...and it takes less than 60 seconds... leave a review.

Simply scan the QR code below to leave your review:

If you feel good about helping someone struggling with their health, you're my kind of person. Welcome to the club.

I'm so excited to help you boost your immune system and manage your condition. You'll love the strategies I'm about to share in the coming chapters.

Thank you from the bottom of my heart. Now, let's get back to learning how to feel your best!

Your biggest fan, Tina Shelton

Chapter 6:

Prolonged Fast and

Nutrition

One of the questions you may have when considering a prolonged fast is how your nutrition would work while you are fasting. Where does your body get the nutrients it needs to survive during a 2-day, 7-day, or 10-day fast? Many people worry that their bodies won't get enough nutrients during this time, and it prevents them from embracing prolonged fasting for improved health, especially if they suffer from chronic conditions that already strain their bodies.

For example, your nutrient absorption is already compromised if you have inflammatory bowel syndrome (IBS). In this case, you may fear that a prolonged fast will lead to malnutrition and associated health conditions. In this chapter, we will discuss how nutrition affects prolonged fasting and how your body receives and processes nutrients during the two stages of fasting.

Nutrition: The Number One Factor of Fasting

Believe it or not, the number one factor of fasting is food intake. The entire principle of fasting is when you eat. Withholding food for certain periods has many health benefits, as discussed in the following chapter. However, while some people become fixated on the idea that fasting is about when you eat, what you eat is also a crucial part of prolonged fasting and can mean the difference between success and failure during a prolonged fast.

As you have seen in previous chapters, consuming certain foods, including refined carbs or carbs in general, immediately after a fast can harm your health and well-being. It can lead to digestive distress and may even cause refeeding syndrome after prolonged fasting. Therefore, while fasting focuses more on when you eat than what you eat, what you eat is also important. Breaking a prolonged fast with refined carbs and processed foods will do more harm than good and will undo all the hard work your body has endured during fasting to improve your health.

When you break a prolonged fast, you really want to focus on foods that will improve your health and increase or utilize the benefits you gained from the fasting period. After a prolonged fast, your body will be in a ketogenic state, as you already know. Ideally, you would want to keep your body in this state for a little longer, leading to increased fat burn, brain health, and gut health. But what does that mean for your diet? Basically, a ketogenic diet is one where your carbohydrate intake is very low, and your fat and protein intake is high. Your body enters ketosis when no glycogen is available for quick energy.

While glycogen is the body's preferred energy source, the body actually does better when it burns fat for energy. In this case, your pancreas and digestive system aren't working as hard to digest the food and regulate your blood glucose levels. If you consume carbohydrates or sugars when breaking a prolonged fast, glucose in the blood will increase, leading to insulin spikes. Insulin spikes may cause refeeding syndrome and lead to diabetes if it is not managed. Therefore, when concluding a prolonged fast, the aim is to remain in a ketogenic state or to introduce foods that will not lead to insulin spikes or place too much strain on the digestive system.

Of course, the foods you eat also impact your health in other ways. Your nutritional intake will be lower if your diet consists primarily of processed foods and refined carbs. For example, while a McDonald's burger has some meat and vegetables, it also has many preservatives, added sugar, and sodium. Therefore, even if this burger makes you feel full, you won't get the nutrients your body needs. Instead, if you really want to make the most of a prolonged fasting regime, you should focus on eating whole foods that are high in nutrients during your eating window. This is not only true for prolonged fasting but for most fasting models.

The difference between other fasting models and prolonged fasting is that your fasting window is much longer. The result is that your body will be more sensitive to the foods you eat. As Dr. Eric Berg (2018) explains, you will become insulin sensitive when prolonged fasting. This means that your body will react to increased blood glucose levels more aggressively, and you will be at greater risk for insulin spikes when breaking a prolonged fast incorrectly. Your body will also respond to nutritionally dense foods a lot better. These foods will help your body restore and replenish its energy reserves much better than processed foods.

All this is to say that what you eat is really important when prolonged fasting. It is the number one way to protect yourself against refeeding syndrome, digestive distress, and other side effects from concluding a prolonged fast. It is also the best way to aid your body in readjusting to food and recovering from the fasting period.

The Two Nutrition Programs: Eating and Fasting

Your body has two nutrition programs that can source nutrients when needed; the eating program and the fasting program. Both of these programs are necessary for optimal health, which is why you must utilize both. When you first start a fasting model, you may notice that you feel extremely hungry at certain times of the day, especially when you would normally eat. That's because your body is used to receiving nutrients at that time.

Your body goes into a sort of autopilot regarding nutrition and energy consumption, and it becomes lazy or unwilling to tap into its other nutrition program if you eat regularly.

Therefore, fasting forces your body to utilize its stored energy, making it less reliant on regular eating times. This leads to overall health and well-being and increases autophagy, human growth hormone, and cellular repair, which are essential processes for chronic disease prevention and management. So, let us now consider your body's two nutrition programs in more detail and how your body accesses and uses these programs to keep you fed and energized.

Eating Program

One of the nutrition programs your body has is an eating program. This is the program your body relies on for nutrients when you are in an eating window. Your body will switch to its eating nutrition program when you break your fast and will continue using this program as its source of nutrients until it has depleted its glycogen stores. This process lasts for around three to four hours after eating. Of course, that depends on the food you eat, the rate of your metabolism, and several other factors. During your body's eating program, it primarily relies on burning glucose for energy.

Glucose is the product of carbohydrates and sugars that the body digests. The body transforms these foods into glucose, which it uses for energy. Any additional glucose that is not needed for energy at that point gets stored for later use. The first energy reserve spot for additional glucose is in the liver, where the energy is ready to be used when you no longer have readily available glucose. When the liver's glucose storages are full, the body stores the additional glucose in other reserves throughout the body, storing it as fat.

Your body prefers using glucose as an energy source, as it is easier to digest. However, using glucose as an energy source is inefficient, as Cynthia Thurlow explains in her *Ted Talk: Intermittent Fasting: Transformational Technique* (2019). People who rely on eating carbohydrates for energy are frequently hungry, they experience intense mood swings, and they often struggle with weight loss and weight management. These factors are caused by the insulin spikes you experience when you consume carbohydrates and sugars for energy, as these foods increase blood glucose levels.

But if your body does not have carbohydrates to use for energy, what will it use? If no glucose reserves are left for your body to use as energy, it will start burning your fat reserves. It takes a lot more energy to burn fat for nutrients, so your body will reach for glucose first. While fat burning takes more energy, people who burn fat for energy are fuller for longer, they have more sustained energy, and they find it easier to lose weight and keep it off (Thurlow, 2019). Their insulin levels won't spike as dramatically when they eat, which can also help prevent many chronic conditions, especially those caused by insulin spikes and higher blood glucose levels.

Therefore, if you want to experience sustained energy and avoid insulin spikes (which could lead to refeeding syndrome) when breaking a fast, you must focus on eating the right foods. Does this mean you cannot eat any carbs at all? No, you can eat carbs. However, choosing low GI carbs, such as brown rice, whole grain pasta and bread, and sweet potatoes, will reduce the insulin spikes you experience when eating these foods. If you want to avoid blood glucose and insulin spikes, it is recommended that you encourage your body to burn fat for energy, which can be done with a ketogenic diet and prolonged fasting.

Fasting Program

Your body's other nutrition program is the fasting program. This is the program your body will rely on when it has depleted its readily available glucose reserves. The first thing that will happen at this time is that your liver will release its stored glucose for your body to use. Once this has been used, your body will enter ketosis. This is the process where it starts burning fat instead of glucose for fuel. Your body can continue burning fat for energy for as long as there are fat reserves to burn or until you break the fast.

Ketones are released by the liver, and they are the metabolic bodies that turn stored fat into energy. Your body typically enters ketosis after about 12 hours of fasting and will continue in this state until it has burned through all your fat reserves or until you break the fast (*Time to Try,* 2020). The great thing about ketosis during fasting is that it gives your digestive system a break. The ketones don't rely on the digestive system to process stored fat and use it for energy. This allows your digestive system to focus on reparation and other processes.

Furthermore, your body can focus on cellular reparation, autophagy, and bundling muscles with HGH that it can build during ketosis. During fasting, your body will produce most of the nutrients required to optimize your health. The nutrients it cannot produce by itself, such as certain minerals and vitamins, you can supplement. You also need to drink enough electrolytes and water to keep your body hydrated. Considering that up to 60% of the human body is water, you must stay hydrated during a prolonged fast to ensure your organs and bodily processes function (Sissons, 2020).

Of course, when you are in a prolonged fasting state, you won't entirely abstain from eating. Certain foods, such as the vegetable soup we discussed in the previous chapter, water, electrolytes, black coffee, tea, and a few other foods, will help you stay satisfied without concluding your fast. We'll discuss these foods and other tips in greater detail in Chapter 9 of this book.

The Importance of Electrolytes While Fasting

You've read the words electrolytes a few times in this book, but we have not yet discussed what electrolytes are and why they are so important for the body, especially when fasting. Since electrolytes form part of your fasting and eating programs, we thought it best to discuss this topic further in this chapter. So, let's consider what electrolytes are, why they are so important for your health, and how prolonged fasting may affect your electrolyte balance.

Why are Electrolytes Important?

An article published in the National Library of Medicine by Shrimanker and Bhattarai (2021) says the following about electrolytes and their importance in our bodies:

> "They carry an electric charge and play a vital role in various organ functions, such as nerve impulses and muscle contractions. Maintaining proper hydration to regulate fluid balance within and outside your cells is crucial. An electrolyte imbalance may cause muscle cramps, dizziness, fatigue, and irregular heartbeats. To restore electrolytes, it's recommended to consume fluids that will help you maintain proper hydration levels before introducing solid foods" (p1).

Electrolytes are substances that can carry an electric charge when they are combined with water. Our bodies absorb electrolytes from food, especially fruits and vegetables. Electrolytes include vital minerals such as sodium, potassium, magnesium, calcium, bicarbonate, phosphorus, and chloride. These electrolytes are responsible for many functions in your body, including the following:

- Electrolytes enable your muscles to contract and relax, which is an important human function.

- Electrolytes help manage your body's pH level, which should be between 7.35 and 7.45.

- Electrolytes help keep you hydrated and are responsible for the exchange of water and waste materials between cells (a process called osmosis).

- Electrolytes support brain functioning. The brain works with electrical charges, which are made possible through the movement of electrolytes.

If your body's electrolytes become depleted or imbalanced, you may experience severe side effects. Electrolyte imbalances may even be fatal if they are not addressed, which is why hydration and proper nutrition are crucial for everyone, even when fasting.

The Role of Electrolytes During Prolonged Fasting

Considering the importance of electrolytes, you may wonder how they are affected by fasting. Despite all the wonderful benefits of prolonged fasting, it carries the risk of your electrolytes becoming depleted or imbalanced. This can lead to several dangerous health complications, including the following:

- headaches

- dizziness

- low blood pressure

- difficulty concentrating

- mood swings and a generally foul mood

- fatigue

- dark urine

- dry skin and cracked lips

- muscle cramps, especially at night

- feeling thirsty all the time

While some of these symptoms are also side effects from fasting, they might indicate that you are dehydrated or that your electrolytes are depleted. Dr. Wiensier (1971) explains that prolonged fasting can cause a loss of vital electrolytes including potassium, sodium, chloride, and magnesium due to sweating and urine production. If your electrolytes are not restored, and you don't drink enough water during a prolonged fast, you may become very ill. You may develop heart arrhythmias and could be hospitalized, or worse, if you don't get yourself rehydrated and replenish your electrolytes. Therefore, you must manage your hydration and electrolyte levels at all times, even during a prolonged fast.

How to Supplement Electrolytes During Prolonged Fasting

Fortunately, even though there is some risk of electrolyte depletion and dehydration when fasting, it is easy enough to prevent this from happening. Drinking plenty of water is the best way to stay hydrated and ensure your electrolytes are balanced during a prolonged fast. Water will help keep you hydrated and ensure proper osmosis. Remember that as you fast, your body enters a detoxing mode where it gets rid of many chemicals and toxins. This leads to frequent urination, which could increase your chances of dehydration. Therefore, you should focus on staying hydrated while fasting.

Furthermore, taking an electrolyte supplement, such as an electrolyte powder, can help manage your electrolyte levels and ensure you stay as healthy and balanced as possible during a prolonged fast. These electrolyte powders usually contain a great blend of minerals that will address any electrolyte imbalances you experience. They are also typically low enough in calories not to break your prolonged fast accidentally.

Dr. Berg (2018) shares another tip for ensuring your electrolytes are balanced before concluding a prolonged fast. He mentions that drinking water with a ¼ teaspoon of baking soda will alkalize your body before concluding a fast. This helps maintain your electrolyte levels and reduces the risk of experiencing any of the side effects mentioned above and the side effects some people experience when breaking a fast.

Finally, eating the right foods, such as dark green vegetables and fresh fruit, adding sodium (not too much) to your food, and taking a magnesium supplement if need be during your eating windows can help maintain healthy electrolyte levels and reduce the risk of electrolyte depletion during a prolonged fast.

Key Takeaway From Chapter 6

Your body has two nutrition programs: one when you are eating and one when you are fasting. Your body will first use any available glucose for energy during your eating program since this is the easiest source. It will also store any additional glucose in the liver and then in fat cells throughout your body. When you are fasting, your body will use all the available glucose reserves first before ultimately switching over to using fat for energy. You will enter ketosis at this time, which will last as long as you have available fat reserves or until you break the fast. Electrolytes are crucial for a healthy body and may become depleted during a prolonged fast. To prevent this from happening, it's important that you stay properly hydrated and consider drinking water with electrolyte powders mixed in to prevent electrolyte depletion.

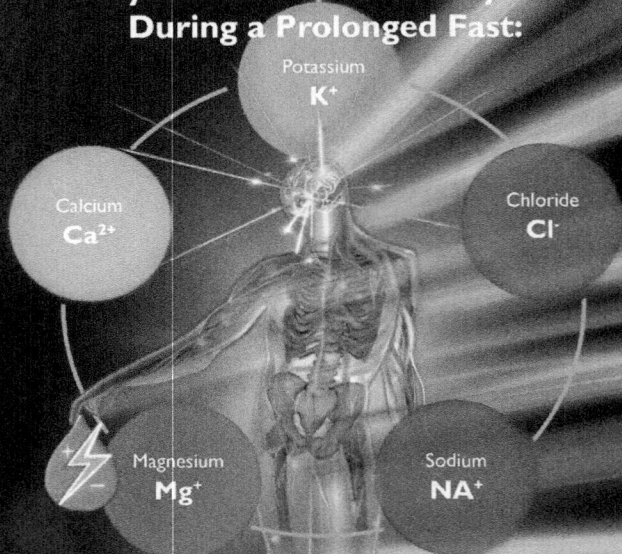

Hydration With Electrolytes During a Prolonged Fast:

Potassium
K^+

Calcium
Ca^{2+}

Chloride
Cl^-

Magnesium
Mg^+

Sodium
NA^+

The Vital Role of Electrolytes:

- help manage your body's pH level

- help keep you hydrated

- responsible for the exchange of water and waste materials between cells

- support brain functioning by creating vital electrical charges through its movement

Chapter 7:

Chronic Diseases and

Prolonged Fasting

Now that we have done an in-depth explanation of prolonged fasting, how it works, and how it can affect your health in general, it is time to explore prolonged fasting and the reason for this book: chronic diseases. We have not been talking about fasting for the past three chapters for no reason. Prolonged fasting and other fasting models have been shown to reduce the effects of chronic conditions on your health significantly. They have also been found to reduce your chances of suffering from chronic conditions, even if you have a genetic risk for them.

Furthermore, fasting has been shown to improve your well-being while undergoing certain treatments, such as chemotherapy. In this chapter, we will consider the effects of prolonged fasting on many chronic diseases and how fasting can improve your diagnosis and quality of life while you overcome them. This is likely one of the book's most insightful and important chapters, so I recommend paying attention, especially when reading about your specific chronic disease or chronic diseases in your family.

Immune System Reset With Prolonged Fasting

According to Cheng et al. (2014), "Prolonged fasting (PF) lasting 48–120 hours reduces pro-growth signaling and activates pathways that enhance cellular resistance to toxins in mice and humans." The research was conducted on mice to determine if prolonged fasting could help repair a compromised immune system. These tests were conducted on two groups of immune-suppressed mice: those undergoing chemotherapy for cancer and those with a compromised immune system because of aging. The results prolonged fasting had on these mice were astonishing, and the fasting protocol may have similar effects on immune-compromised humans.

Fasting showed improvements for patients undergoing chemotherapy for cancer. Chemotherapy compromises a person's immune system because of the damage it causes to the cells in the body. While this helps shrink cancerous cells, it also damages healthy ones. As such, it severely affects your immune system, which can take a long time to recover even after the chemotherapy has concluded. We'll discuss the effects of fasting on chemotherapy and cancer patients in greater detail in the following section. For now, though, it is worth noting that studies conducted on mice showed significant improvements in the immune system of the mice that received chemotherapy treatments.

You won't only have a compromised immune system when undergoing chemotherapy. In fact, something as simple as aging can also cause a compromised immune system. As you get older, cellular regeneration slows down. It takes longer for damaged and dying cells to be replaced. This affects your immune system, as the organs and glands that keep you healthy may start to deteriorate. You may become immune-compromised, and non-threatening illnesses like a common cold can make you severely ill.

Fortunately, the same research conducted on mice to determine the effects of fasting on chemotherapy patients was also conducted on mice that were immune compromised because of aging. And just like in the case of the chemotherapy immune-compromised chemotherapy mice, the mice with compromised immune systems because of aging also experienced significant improvements in their immune systems when practicing prolonged fasting (Cheng et al., 2014). This could mean greater health benefits for older people, especially those with compromised immune systems or those who may experience a compromised immune system after surgery, illness, or treatment.

But how exactly does prolonged fasting assist with resetting the immune system? It starts in the bone marrow, where hematopoietic stem cells (HSC) are created. These hematopoietic stem cells consist of marrow and blood cells, crucial for a stronger immune system. These are some of the first cells to get damaged during chemotherapy and aging, so these conditions often lead to a compromised immune system. However, prolonged fasting improves hematopoietic stem cell production in mice undergoing chemotherapy and those immuno-compromised because of aging (Cheng et al., 2014). By increasing HSC production, your body will have a stronger immune system, helping it fight infections, chemo-toxicity, and some chronic conditions related to a compromised immune system.

Prolonged fasting can, therefore, improve your immune system and reset it. There are so many factors, apart from aging and chemotherapy, that affect your immune system. Lifestyle choices, such as diet, exercise, harmful habits (smoking and frequent drinking), pollution, medicine, and the general environment, have become counter-productive to building a stronger immune system. People are exposed to many pollutants, including chronic stress, which severely affects their immune system, placing more stress on their bodies and potentially leading to a compromised immune system.

Of course, many foods we eat, especially highly processed foods and sugary foods, also attack our immune systems and introduce many unwanted chemicals to our bodies, which our immune system is responsible for disposing of. Therefore, a prolonged fast that cleanses your body of all these collected pathogens and chemicals also helps your immune system. It can reset your immune system and increase your HSC levels to optimal levels. By resetting your immune system, you can improve your overall health and well-being, helping to prevent and manage several chronic conditions.

If you think about it, your immune system significantly affects your health. So, by helping build a stronger immune system, prolonged fasting indirectly affects your health in many ways. For example, many people have found relief from autoimmune diseases, such as arthritis, rheumatism, IBS, and more, from prolonged fasting. But fasting also has a much more direct impact on certain other health conditions, including cancer. Let's consider how prolonged fasting can help you beat and prevent cancer.

Beat and Prevent Cancer With Prolonged Fasting

Since cancer is a big concern for many people, and it is one of the most common chronic conditions, considering how prolonged fasting may help prevent or combat cancer has been a topic of interest for many researchers. There are so many factors that cause and contribute to cancer. While your genes play a role in your risk of developing certain types of cancer, these risks are only increased by our way of life. Unfortunately, many things we use daily contain materials or substances that are known carcinogens or cancer-causing materials.

Carcinogens are substances with a known cancer-causing risk. There are carcinogens all around us. For example, the ultraviolet light emitted by the sun is a physical carcinogen, as it may increase your risk of skin cancer. Formaldehyde and melamine are carcinogenic substances found in most plastic products, including plastic cutlery, crockery, and toys. Certain infections are also carcinogens, as are certain pollutants you find around your home daily.

Therefore, it can be extremely difficult to determine the cause of your cancer or mitigate the risk entirely with lifestyle changes and diet. But the good news is that prolonged fasting can help you beat and prevent cancer, not only because it strengthens your immune system, allowing your body to fight cancer by itself, but also because it causes many cancer-fighting functions in the body. So, how does prolonged fasting help prevent and beat cancer?

One way fasting helps prevent cancer is by reducing your IGF-1 hormone. IGF-1 stands for Insulin-like Growth Hormone type 1 (Berg, 2020). IGF-1 functions just like HGH and is a vital hormone during fasting. HGH is produced in the pituitary gland in the brain. It then travels to the liver, where IGF-1 is produced. IGF-1, like HGH, is responsible for tissue growth and tissue production. IGF-1 is also responsible for mobilizing fat for energy while you are fasting. When you are fasting, your IGF-1 levels tend to increase.

Unfortunately, while IGF-1 is crucial for tissue growth and fat mobilization, it has also been linked to cancer. Because IGF-1 causes tissue growth, it may also cause cancerous cells to grow, as many other growth hormones in the body do. Moreover, IGF-1 inhibits apoptosis, which is a crucial process that occurs in the body. Apoptosis causes many biochemical changes in the body, which causes cell death or cell suicide in cells it perceives as a threat, such as cancerous cells. So, IGF-1 causes increased tissue growth while inhibiting cellular death. But if IGF-1 increases your risk of cancer, and these levels rise when fasting, how does prolonged fasting help prevent cancer?

Dr. Eric Berg (2020) states that your IGF-1 levels decrease after fasting for 3 to 5 days. Your IGF-1 levels will decrease by around 30% at this time. And if you fast for longer than 5 days, you may notice a 60% decrease in IGF-1 while HGH levels continue to increase. You will also experience a significant drop in blood glucose and insulin levels. All these factors create an environment in your body where cancer cells cannot survive. Therefore, a prolonged fast is a great way to prevent cancer by creating an inhospitable environment in your body.

Another way prolonged fasting can reduce your cancer risk is by increasing autophagy. As you already know, autophagy is when your body digests damaged and dead cells to repair other cells. The interesting part of prolonged fasting, as explained by Longo and Mattson (2014), is that autophagy works in combination with apoptosis. When you are fasting, your body destroys any unwanted cells. Then, during the refeeding period (after breaking a fast), your body will work extremely hard to replace those destroyed cells with healthy ones.

In an interview, Dr. Valter Longo also explains that prolonged fasting can help prevent cancer by causing differential stress resistance (Patrick, 2016). This is a condition where the healthy cells become resistant to stress in the body, while cancer cells cannot thrive or grow under these conditions. Furthermore, prolonged fasting may lead to differential stress sensitization, where the cancer cells are more sensitive to cell death because of the stress your body is under while the healthy cells survive.

According to Dr. Longo, when fasting, your healthy cells enter a "protected mode," which becomes much more resistant to stress and toxicity while waiting for food. On the contrary, cancer cells cannot enter a protective mode during fasting, as they rely on cellular changes to keep growing. This means that your cancer cells will starve and die while your healthy cells stay in their protected mode. As such, prolonged fasting improves your body's resistance to stress and kills off cancerous cells before they can multiply and grow.

If you have already been diagnosed with cancer and are undergoing treatment, such as chemotherapy, you may wonder if prolonged fasting can provide any benefit in this case. Let's consider how prolonged fasting can improve your health if you undergo cancer treatments and how fasting may prevent cancer from reoccurring.

Fasting for Chemotherapy: Practical Advice

If you undergo chemotherapy, you are likely already very ill. Not only has your cancer progressed to a stage where chemotherapy is necessary to kill the cells, but you are also experiencing chemo toxicity, which causes massive cell deaths of healthy cells in your body. As you already know, this also significantly affects your immune system and can put you at risk of contracting secondary infections. Therefore, you may wish to do everything possible to keep your body healthy during chemotherapy. And you may wonder how prolonged fasting can be beneficial if you are already undergoing chemotherapy or if it is worth considering.

Fasting for Prevention or Reoccurrence

Cancer cells have always been considered very smart. However, Dr. Longo explains in his interview with Dr. Rhonda Patric (2016) that cancer cells are actually not that smart at all. He explains that cancer cells typically grow and multiply in nutrient-rich environments, feeding on sugars (glucose) and amino acids. And while the other cells in your body are conditioned to live off fat cells during fasting, the cancer cells cannot effectively digest and utilize fat cells. Therefore, if you are fasting, your healthy cells continue to get the nutrients they need from another source, while the cancer cells essentially starve and are then destroyed by apoptosis.

This means that fasting is one way to prevent cancer from growing in your body. It can also, therefore, be used as a way to prevent cancer from reoccurring. Doing a prolonged fast once a month will enable your body to deal with stress much better, and you will prevent cancer cells from thriving in your body. While prolonged fasting can be extremely beneficial in cancer prevention, it does put a lot of strain on your body. As such, it is recommended that you perform a prolonged fast under medical supervision, especially if you are recovering from cancer, have recently been diagnosed with cancer, or have an increased risk of cancer.

Fasting When You Have Cancer

The standard treatment method for cancer patients includes parental nutrition, which is nutrition you receive through your veins or means other than your mouth. However, according to Dr. Micheal Gregor (2023), cancer cells act like a fetus in a pregnant woman, and they prioritize themselves and their needs when you receive any nutrients, regardless of your overall health. This is why many cancer patients' weight declines even when given hundreds of additional calories daily. Dr. Gregor also mentions that perhaps the reason why cancer patients lose their appetite is because the body is trying to starve those cancer cells.

As discussed in the previous section, healthy cells can enter a survive and repair or protection mode when you don't eat. Cancer cells cannot do this because they rely on nutrients, specifically glucose, to grow and mutate. This means that fasting might not be such a new concept to introduce to cancer patients as many of us think. Your loss of appetite might be your body's way of naturally inducing fasting to help you fight against cancer. And many studies have proven just how effective fasting can be, particularly in combination with chemotherapy.

For example, one study found that a 24-48 hour fast before chemotherapy resulted in the chemotherapy drugs having a 24% increase in effect (Gregor, 2023). Prolonged fasting, therefore, reduces the growth of cancer cells and helps make the cancer treatment more effective. An additional benefit of fasting while undergoing chemotherapy is that your healthy cells are protected against the effects of chemo toxicity. This will help to prevent secondary infection, improve your quality of life, and improve your chance of survival.

Furthermore, fasting during chemotherapy can also improve your immune system, which might help reduce the side effects you experience from the treatment. Make no mistake; chemotherapy poisons your body, and there have been instances where patients have died from the effects of chemotherapy on their weakened bodies (Gregor, 2023). While chemotherapy was initially thought to only attack the cancerous cells, it has since been discovered that cancer also affects healthy cells and can cause cell death among healthy cells. Therefore, even if prolonged fasting only benefits your immune system (which it does not), it would still be worthwhile considering it as a therapy while undergoing cancer treatment.

One thing to note about fasting during cancer treatment, as noted by Dr. Wilhelmi de Toledo, is that all human clinical studies where fasting was prescribed as a treatment had a much greater effect on the patients who embraced prolonged fasting as a therapy (Wilhelmi de Toledo, 2022). Patients who voluntarily embraced fasting as therapy and believed it could help them showed much greater results than those forced to embrace prolonged fasting as part of the study. Furthermore, Dr. Wilhelmi de Toledo pointed out that it is crucial to discuss prolonged fasting as a treatment method with your oncologist and other doctors to ensure everyone is on the same page.

Once you have gotten the all-clear from your doctors, you can discuss your fasting protocol with a prolonged fasting specialist. They will recommend the ideal fasting plan based on your circumstances. Your type of cancer, current weight, overall health, and mental state will affect the type of prolonged fasting plan recommended for you. While fasting has many benefits for the body, you must recognize that your body is weakened from cancer and chemotherapy. Therefore, clinical observation is crucial when committing to prolonged fasting, as you will be more affected by certain changes during fasting.

Beat and Prevent Heart Disease With Prolonged Fasting

Fasting has significant effects on cancer and your general health while undergoing cancer treatments, such as chemotherapy. But cancer is not the only chronic condition where prolonged fasting may prove an effective treatment. Fasting has also been shown to help you beat and prevent heart disease, another common chronic condition affecting many's duration and quality of life. Let's consider how fasting can help beat and prevent heart disease.

One way in which prolonged fasting can help prevent heart disease is by forcing your cells into a protected state, where they focus on repair. This means that prolonged fasting can increase your heart health by repairing any damaged cells that may lead to cardiac diseases, including heart attacks. By increasing autophagy, prolonged fasting increases cellular regeneration throughout your body and heart. This means that the damaged cells and tissue, which may cause heart conditions, are replaced and repaired, reducing your chances of heart disease.

Another way in which prolonged fasting can help prevent and beat heart disease is by managing your weight. The more body mass you have, the harder your heart must work to pump blood throughout your body. This puts a lot of strain on your heart. And, after many years of being under such immense pressure, your heart may start failing. However, since prolonged fasting induces a ketogenic state, during which fat cells are burned for energy, it can help you lose weight and keep it off. This relieves some of the pressure on your heart and can prevent it from failing altogether.

In addition, by consuming fat reserves for energy, your body may also burn any fatty deposits that gather in your arteries. These fatty deposits form in your arteries if you overeat fatty or processed foods. They can potentially cause heart failure, a heart attack, or stroke. But as your body requires more fat to burn for energy during a prolonged fast, these fatty deposits will also be reduced. In this way, prolonged fasting can help prevent a heart attack.

Yet another way in which fasting can prevent and beat heart disease is by balancing your cholesterol levels. Research has found that fasting can help reduce LDL cholesterol and increase HDL cholesterol levels (Lopez-Jimenez, 2022). Since high LDL levels are associated with several heart conditions, prolonged fasting can help manage your health by managing these cholesterol levels.

Furthermore, as you already know, prolonged fasting can reduce blood glucose levels and, therefore, manage insulin levels. By doing so, prolonged fasting helps to regulate the glucose in your blood, which can assist with weight management and decrease your chances of developing diabetes, which is a significant risk factor for heart disease.

One study was conducted to determine the effects of fasting on lifespan following a cardiac catheterization procedure (*Regular Fasting*, 2019). This is a procedure where a doctor runs a thin tube through an artery into your heart to run certain diagnostic tests. It is often performed on people with cardiac disease, and a similar procedure is often used to open blocked arteries in the case of heart disease. This study was done on a Mormon population, who typically fast for 24 hours or one Sunday a month. While this is not really considered prolonged fasting, it sheds some light on what effects prolonged fasting may have on heart disease.

The research concluded that Mormons who routinely fasted post-cardiac catheterization experienced a 45% lower mortality rate than those who did not practice fasting (*Regular Fasting*, 2019). Furthermore, routine fasters had a 71% reduced chance of developing heart disease than those who did not routinely fast. This evidence suggests a strong possibility that fasting can improve your heart health, helping to beat and prevent heart conditions and cardiac disease.

Another study considered the effects of fasting on a 64-year-old male admitted to the hospital with angina and exertional dyspnea (shortness of breath). After being recommended he had surgery, the patient refused treatment and placed himself on a 50-day water fast instead (Gajagowni et al., 2022). While the man was hospitalized during this fasting period for dehydration, his cardiac symptoms improved to the point where surgery was no longer necessary. After concluding the 50-day fast, the patient continued with a high-protein vegan diet and intermittent fasting and has not complained of heart health since.

While these studies are mere examples of small-scale effects of prolonged fasting on heart health, they strongly indicate that it can improve heart health and prevent heart disease. Even if the effects of prolonged fasting are only that it aids in weight loss and insulin management, that is still reason enough to consider it as a treatment method and preventative measure for heart conditions.

Beat and Prevent Stroke With Prolonged Fasting

Since strokes are another common chronic condition that severely affects your quality of life, and considering how the previous book focused on the effects of fasting on brain health, you may wonder if prolonged fasting can reduce your risk of getting a stroke. According to the World Stroke Association, 25% of the global population experiences a stroke at least once in their life (*Learn About Stroke*, n.d.). A stroke is a condition that occurs in your brain when something (fat, blood clots, or other materials) blocks an artery in a part of the brain or if an artery in the brain ruptures. Strokes can be fatal, or they may cause long-term damage, such as slurred speech, partial paralysis, memory loss, personality changes, or more. The damage caused by a stroke depends on where in the brain the stroke occurs.

Regardless of where a stroke occurs or how severe it is, strokes are scary for the people experiencing them and those around them. Furthermore, as strokes can cause lasting effects, it is worth considering how you can reduce your chances of stroke. While strokes are not always caused by genetics, there is a genetic component to it. If your family members tend to have high blood pressure, high cholesterol, or a history of stroke, you are at greater risk for having a stroke yourself. So, what does the research suggest about the effects of prolonged fasting on stroke?

Animal studies have shown that fasting can reduce the brain damage caused by a stroke and improve the functional recovery of the brain and the body after a stroke (Phillips, 2019). These studies, while conducted on animals, may prove true for humans as well. Why is this? There are several reasons why prolonged fasting can reduce the damage caused to the brain during a stroke. One of the reasons is that fasting sends the body's cells into protection mode, where they focus on recovery. This factor occurs throughout the body, including in the brain. In a way, this also conditions the brain somewhat, making it more resistant to stress.

Another reason fasting may reduce a stroke's effects on your brain and body is that fasting is known to reduce inflammation (Phillips, 2019). Inflammation is one of the leading causes of stroke and can result from weight gain, stress, and poor lifestyle choices and diet. By reducing inflammation throughout the body, fasting helps prevent plaque buildup in the brain's arteries. Plaque is a build-up of protein fragments and other materials that gather in the artery walls. This build-up can cause a narrowing of the arteries and may lead to a blockage, which can cause a stroke.

However, fasting can help prevent this plaque build-up by preventing inflammation in the arteries. This can also prevent a stroke by keeping the arteries in the brain healthy. Another way fasting can help reduce the effects of a stroke on your brain and body is by reducing your chances of heart disease. Heart disease is closely connected with brain health, and people with heart disease are automatically at greater risk for stroke. But as you know from the previous section, fasting has many significant health benefits for your heart and can help prevent and beat heart disease, thereby reducing your chances of stroke.

Prolonged or intermittent fasting in mice has also proven effective in helping the brain heal after a stroke and improving your survival chances (Chelluboina et al., 2020). This study compared mice that experienced intermittent fasting before a stroke with those that ate regular meals. Not only did the mice that fasted before the stroke experience fewer side effects, but they also recovered faster and better than the mice that did not experience fasting. Several tests, such as walking on a beam and rotarod tests, were used to compare the study groups regarding motor skills and recovery. Furthermore, these studies showed that the fasted mice had a higher post-stroke survival rate of 80% than the non-fasted mice, which only had a survival rate of 40%. This shows that fasting may also improve your chances of survival after a severe stroke.

A similar study that also used mice to determine the effects of fasting on stroke concluded that fasting after traumatic brain injury or stroke helps protect the brain and increase recovery. This study also mentioned that "It is likely that upregulated BDNF, enhanced mitochondria function, activated stress response signaling pathways, and suppressed neuroinflammation also play important roles" (Phillips, 2019). These benefits all result from fasting, too. Book 2 in this series has a detailed explanation of the effects of fasting on brain health and the role of BDNF in improving brain health and preventing stroke.

Beat and Prevent Diabetes With Prolonged Fasting

Since we've mentioned insulin levels a few times, you may wonder how fasting can help prevent or beat diabetes. As you may know, there are different kinds of diabetes, and each type has different outcomes and treatment methods. Whatever type of diabetes you have, fasting may provide some benefits to curing the condition or at least reducing your symptoms.

Diabetes is caused when your blood sugar levels are too high or your body cannot produce enough insulin to manage the raised blood sugar levels. Some medication is usually required to manage blood glucose and insulin levels. However, based on what you already know from previous chapters, prolonged fasting affects your blood glucose and insulin levels. Let's consider how fasting can affect these levels to help beat and prevent diabetes.

Type 1 Diabetes and Prolonged Fasting

Type 1 diabetes, also known as insulin-dependent diabetes, is a chronic condition that affects your pancreas. It causes your pancreas to stop producing insulin either entirely or to a great extent, meaning you must take chemical insulin, usually in the form of injections. Type-1 diabetes is a genetic condition, meaning you are at greater risk if someone in your family has it. This type of diabetes usually makes itself known during childhood or early adolescence and requires life-long treatment. There is no known cure for type-1 diabetes at the moment. But what does that mean for prolonged fasting?

While prolonged fasting may not be able to cure type-1 diabetes, it certainly can improve your quality of life and reduce your insulin dependence. What happens when you have type-1 diabetes is that you become more sensitive to the foods you eat. Since your body doesn't produce its own insulin and you are reliant on a metered dose of insulin, foods that minimally affect other people's blood glucose levels may cause yours to spike significantly. Determining how much insulin you need also depends on what you eat, when you eat, and your blood glucose levels before administering the insulin.

This means that if you can control your blood glucose levels, you can reduce the amount of insulin your body needs, meaning you won't need as large a dose of insulin to stay healthy. Fasting, both intermittent and prolonged fasting, reduces your blood glucose levels and your need for insulin. Prolonged fasting can alter how your body uses fuel (reaching for fats instead of glucose), helping to monitor your blood glucose levels even when you are not fasting. These effects are increased if you combine prolonged fasting with a ketogenic diet that limits the amount of carbs and sugars you consume.

However, even though prolonged fasting may improve type-1 diabetes, Dr. Jody Stalinslaw (2022) explains that you should only consider prolonged fasting if you are confident with dosing your insulin correctly. By this, she means that since you will no longer consume carbs or foods that may cause blood glucose spikes, your insulin dose must be adjusted. If you don't adjust your insulin properly, your blood sugar levels may go too low, leading to seizures, coma, or even death. Therefore, if you are considering prolonged fasting for type-1 diabetes, it is recommended that you consult with your healthcare provider first and learn how to adjust your insulin dose correctly.

Type 2 Diabetes and Prolonged Fasting

Unlike type-1 diabetes, type-2 diabetes means that your body cannot properly use the insulin it produces. While there are cases in which your body simply does not produce enough insulin to counteract the glucose in your blood, other times, the insulin simply isn't used correctly by the body. Your risk for type-2 diabetes, like type-1, can increase based on your genetics. Type-2 diabetes is curable in many cases, and it can develop at any age. Type-2 diabetes can also occur because of poor lifestyle choices, including living a sedentary lifestyle, a diet filled with refined carbs and processed foods, smoking, and stress. However, lifestyle choices aren't always the cause of type-2 diabetes.

On a positive note, prolonged fasting, or even intermittent fasting, can help reduce the effects of type-2 diabetes on your health and well-being. It might actually be able to prevent and beat type-2 diabetes under the right circumstances. Depending on the severity of your type-2 diabetes, you may be able to manage it simply by making some lifestyle changes. In other cases, you may be required to take some medications to manage your insulin and blood glucose levels. Let's consider how fasting can help reduce type-2 diabetes and possibly even cure it.

The primary way in which fasting can help manage and prevent type-2 diabetes is by reducing your blood glucose levels. Dr. Eric Berg (2013) states that your blood glucose levels should be around 100 mg/dL. If your blood glucose levels drop too far below this mark, you will enter hypoglycemia, which can cause various health conditions, including seizures and coma. Suppose your blood glucose levels rise too high above this mark. In that case, your body might not produce enough insulin to manage it, and you may become hyperglycemic, which can also cause various health conditions and might even be fatal. So, the ideal is to remain around the 100 mg/DL mark.

Fasting can help to keep you at this mark by reducing the glucose in your blood. As you already know, when you are fasting, your body burns stored fat for energy, which causes a decrease in blood glucose levels and fewer insulin spikes. This can prevent or even treat type-2 diabetes if administered early enough after detection. Prolonged fasting, or even intermittent fasting combined with a low-carb or ketogenic, can significantly reduce your chances of developing type-2 diabetes. As such, it will be greatly beneficial to start this diet as soon as possible, especially if your doctor has warned you about having an increased risk of developing type-2 diabetes.

Of course, you should also consult your doctor before starting a prolonged fast, especially if you are on insulin medication. Do not attempt a prolonged fast against your doctor's advice if it is regarding your medication. In this case, shorter intermittent fasting models, such as a 14/6 or 12/12 fast, may be better suited to your needs. However, a diabetic specialist and diabetic specialist nutritionist should be able to give you much more detailed information regarding the suitable fasting models and overall nutrition if you have type-2 diabetes.

Beat and Prevent IBS With Prolonged Fasting

While we haven't really discussed the influence of fasting on gut health in previous chapters, you can find an in-depth explanation of all the benefits of fasting for gut health and the best fasting protocols for gut health in the first book of this series. I would like to focus on one chronic disease that affects your gut and can be improved with prolonged fasting. Irritable Bowel Syndrome (IBS) is a chronic condition affecting around 15% of the earth's population, with women being at greater risk (*The Statistics of*, n.d.).

IBS is an inflammatory disease that causes intestinal distress. Common factors of IBS include bloating, indigestion, nausea, vomiting, diarrhea, and constipation. IBS is a chronic condition and often requires lifelong management. Unfortunately, there is no cure for IBS at this moment. But how can prolonged fasting help with treating or managing this disease? According to Dr. Ryan Warren (Lindberg, 2019), intermittent fasting may help to activate the Migrating Motor Complex (MMC), which helps move food along the intestinal tract. An inactive MMC has been connected to SIBO, an overgrowth of bacteria in the small intestine, which is often at fault for causing IBS.

Another way prolonged fasting can help improve symptoms of IBS is by giving the digestive tract a break. If you are constantly eating at short intervals, your digestive system is placed under a lot of stress to digest and process the foods. And if these foods are difficult to digest, your intestines are under even more pressure. This might also be the cause of your IBS. But if you endure a prolonged fast, your entire digestive tract gets a break, allowing your digestive system to repair itself and replace damaged cells.

If you conclude the prolonged fast, your digestive system will be renewed, and it can digest the food much easier and more effectively. Furthermore, prolonged fasting activates autophagy, which helps repair any damaged cells in your digestive system. Prolonged fasting is also related to decreased inflammation, which is another significant contributor to IBS. Therefore, prolonged or intermittent fasting may help reduce your IBS symptoms while also helping to treat the disease in the long term.

However, Dr. Warren also mentions that prolonged fasting might not be an effective treatment in all cases of IBS, as breaking a fast may lead to overeating and place more stress on the digestive system during that time. Therefore, it's crucial to start with small, easily digestible meals when concluding a fast to help your digestive system get used to processing food and nutrients again. Furthermore, if you are sensitive or intolerant to certain foods, you may still have to avoid them even if you are fasting, as these foods may still trigger an IBS flare-up if you consume them during your eating window.

Key Takeaway From Chapter 7

Prolonged and Intermittent fasting has many proven benefits for combating and preventing certain chronic conditions, including heart disease, stroke, and type-2 diabetes. Prolonged fasting may also relieve the symptoms of type-1 diabetes, helping to reduce your insulin dependency. Furthermore, prolonged fasting has astonishing benefits in cancer prevention and can protect cells against chemo toxicity during chemotherapy. Prolonged fasting can also act as a type of immune system reset, which can help strengthen your immune system, thereby making your body more resistant to chronic disease and secondary infections. Prolonged fasting also has some benefits for IBS and can help manage this chronic disease.

Chronically Ill Body Before and During a Prolonged Fast (PF):

Before PF:

Proliferation of damaged cells e.g. cancerous cells
- immune system compromised
- body prone to infection, chemo-toxicity and more chronic diseases

Reduced production of hematopoietic stem cells (HSC), which are responsible for immune system reset

Apoptosis, autophagy processes are compromised

Poor weight management may impact on health

Fatty deposits and plaque gathered in arteries may potentially lead to heart disease and stroke

Increased body inflammation

Inactive MMC (Migrating Motor Complex) may lead to IBS, e.g. SIBO

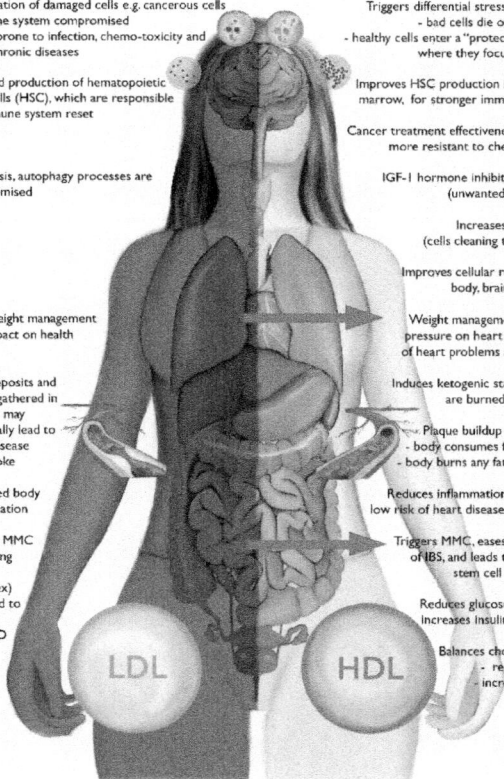

During PF:

Triggers differential stress resistance:
- bad cells die of starvation
- healthy cells enter a "protected" mode, where they focus on repair

Improves HSC production in the bone marrow, for stronger immune system

Cancer treatment effectiveness e.g. cells more resistant to chemotherapy

IGF-1 hormone inhibits apoptosis (unwanted cell death)

Increases autophagy (cells cleaning themselves)

Improves cellular repair in the body, brain and heart

Weight management relieves pressure on heart (lower risk of heart problems and stroke)

Induces ketogenic state: fat cells are burned for energy

Plaque buildup prevention:
- body consumes fat reserves
- body burns any fatty deposits

Reduces inflammation, leading to low risk of heart disease and stroke

Triggers MMC, eases symptoms of IBS, and leads to intestinal stem cell production

Reduces glucose levels and increases insulin sensitivity

Balances cholesterol by
- reducing LDL
- increasing HDL

LDL

HDL

Chapter 8:

Into the Science of Fasting

and Chronic Disease

While it's easy to talk about the effects of fasting on chronic disease based on my own experience and stories I have heard (we'll share more about that in Chapter 10), many of you may wonder if there is any scientific evidence to back these claims up. So many holistic and alternative therapies make amazing claims to heal all kinds of diseases, but they aren't based on scientific research or evidence. Sometimes, these therapies may even be counterproductive and make you sicker. Therefore, it's only natural that you may have questions regarding the validity of prolonged fasting for chronic disease, especially as some of our shared advice goes against current medical trends, such as restricting calories during chemotherapy.

In this chapter, we will consider the research that has been done to support the effects of prolonged and intermittent fasting on chronic disease. We will consider the leading researchers in this field and their research, what scientific evidence there is to back the claims we have made in previous chapters, and the results of these studies. We will also consider how the research may continue or change in the future to give us more information and a tailored fasting and nutrition approach to combating chronic disease.

What Scientific Evidence is There for Fasting (PF and IF)?

Many of you may wonder about the scientific evidence for prolonged and intermittent fasting and how it relates to improvement in chronic diseases. This is a valid question, and I am very interested in it. Fortunately, there are brilliant minds at work in the field of chronic disease and fasting. They have dedicated years of their lives to studying the effects of various fasting protocols on chronic disease.

They have also conducted studies to determine if fasting negatively affects people with chronic diseases and how to mitigate these effects. Let's consider some of the most prominent researchers in the field of fasting and chronic disease and what their research has discovered.

Leading Professionals in the Field of Prolonged Fasting and Chronic Conditions

While there are many professionals in the field of fasting and chronic disease, a few names stand out from the crowd. This is not an exhaustive list and is limited because of language constraints. However, these are three of the leading researchers in this field and people whose research I personally have studied extensively for personal gain and when writing this book. Whether you seek practical advice or in-depth clinical studies, these researchers can help you on your fasting journey. Here are three of the top minds in the field of fasting and chronic disease.

Dr. Valter Longo

Doctor Valter Longo is an Italian-American biologist specializing in studying cell biology and the effects of fasting on cellular responses. Dr. Longo has made significant progress in understanding how prolonged fasting affects the body, specifically how it affects cancerous and aging cells. What's fascinating about Dr. Longo's work is that he studies the effects of fasting on various organisms, from single-celled organisms such as yeast to complex organisms such as mice. Dr. Longo has also applied his research to human studies to understand if the same results found in animals and simple organisms can also be found in humans.

Through his studies, Dr. Longo has discovered that fasting might be a more natural state than we think. The body may promote an atmosphere for fasting when it is ill by reducing or removing your appetite to put you in a fasting state. This suggests that the brain and body may know of the positive effects of fasting in combating and curing chronic diseases. Dr. Longo has made significant progress in understanding how prolonged fasting can prevent cancer and cancer cells from growing and increase the body's resistance to chemo toxicity.

Dr. Eric Berg

Dr. Eric Berg is an American Chiropractic doctor specializing in ketosis and fasting. Dr. Berg believes that fasting can cure many, if not most, chronic and acute conditions. While he believes in the effects of many fasting models, he often focuses on intermittent and prolonged fasting. Dr. Eric Berg is most famous for his informative and easy-to-follow YouTube videos, which explain the intricate details of fasting and ketosis, including the effects fasting has on your body. Dr. Berg has also written several books on the topic for which he has done extensive research.

With his simple and informative YouTube videos, Dr. Berg has been able to help many people understand the effects of fasting on their bodies and how they can use different fasting models for improved health and well-being. He also makes videos explaining practical topics, such as "common fasting mistakes" and "best foods to eat when breaking a fast," to give his viewers all the necessary information to improve their health with fasting while practicing all the necessary safety measures when doing so. Dr. Berg has made information about fasting accessible and easily understandable to many, which is why he is such a prominent figure in this field.

Dr. Otto Buchinger and the Buchinger Wilhelmi Clinic

Dr. Otto Buchinger is the founder of the Buchinger Wilhelmi Clinics in Germany. He started the first clinic in 1953. The clinic is still owned and run by his family, and it is now in the capable hands of the 4th generation of the Buchinger-Wilhelmi family. Under Dr. Otto's and his descendants' guidance, the Buchinger Wilhelmi clinic has been a forerunner in studying the effects of prolonged fasting on many chronic diseases. The clinics offer a place for people to come and partake in prolonged fasting under strict clinical supervision.

Guests who attend the clinic can try prolonged fasting for a set period, usually of about 10 days. The clinic has doctors, chefs, nutritionists, physiotherapists, and personal trainers on staff to ensure their guests are safe and in prime health while undergoing the fast. Through the years, the Buchinger Wilhelmi Clinic has made some interesting discoveries and breakthroughs in understanding how fasting affects the body and how it can improve your health and reduce or even cure some chronic diseases. While the clinic focuses on therapy instead of research, its techniques are based on scientific evidence and the works of Dr. Otto Buchinger and various other medical professionals who have studied fasting intensely.

Studies Conducted to Determine the Effects of Prolonged and Intermittent Fasting on Chronic Conditions

Now that you are familiar with some of the most prominent figures in the field let's consider the research they have done that contributed to the field of chronic conditions and fasting. Much of this research has proved valuable for understanding fasting and how it affects the body. Through their research, we have gained insights into how the body reacts to fasting, which processes fasting enhances and inhibits, and how you can improve your fasting and eating habits for increased results and benefits while fasting. This research has been a critical turning point in the medical and scientific communities and has helped many who were skeptical about fasting as a therapy for chronic disease change their opinions and at least admit that there could be some benefit. So, let's see what the research entailed and what it showed.

Dr. Valter Longo published a study with Mark P. Mattson in *Science Direct* (2014), titled *Fasting: Molecular Mechanisms and Clinical Applications,* where they discussed the research they had done on mice and other organisms to determine the effects of prolonged fasting on cancerous and aging cells. Their research yielded fascinating results in both simple organisms, such as E.coli, and mammals, such as mice. They made the following observation in their study (Longo & Mattson, 2014):

> "Studies of animals show robust and applicable effects of fasting on health indicators including greater insulin sensitivity and reduced levels of

blood pressure, body fat, IGF-I, insulin, glucose, atherogenic lipids, and inflammation. Fasting regimens can ameliorate disease processes and improve functional outcomes in animal models of disorders that include cancer, myocardial infarction, diabetes, stroke, AD, and PD" (p.36).

We'll discuss their results and what the evidence shows for humans in the following section. Another observational study by Andreas Michalsen and Chenying Li, titled *Fasting Therapy for Treating and Preventing Disease - Current State of Evidence* (2013), yielded similar results as the study published by Longo and Mattson. They noted that fasting yields beneficial effects for several health conditions, including chronic conditions, and that more data and research are needed to study these effects further. They also noted the following in their study (Michalsen & Chenying, 2013):

"Various identified mechanisms of fasting point to its potential health-promoting effects. For example, increased production of neurotrophic factors, fasting-induced neuroendocrine activation and hormetic stress response, reduced mitochondrial oxidative stress, general decrease of signs related to aging, and increased autophagy" (p.1).

Yet another study published in the *National Library of Medicine* by the authors Guillaume Fond, Alexandra Macgregor, Marion Leboyer, and Andreas Michalsen, titled *Fasting in Mood Disorders: Neurobiology and Effectiveness. A literature review* (2013) investigated the effects of fasting on mental health and mood improvement. Their article focused on exploring the aspects of prolonged fasting that could have an impact on brain function concerning mood. What's interesting about this study is that it combines the physical and mental aspects of prolonged and intermittent fasting. Seeing as anxiety and depression statistics are alarmingly high, one can consider these disorders to be chronic illnesses as well. The application of fasting models on mental health conditions may prove to be an invaluable resource for overcoming and managing these disorders, giving fasting yet another foot to stand on.

While there are many more research articles and studies to review, these examples should show that fasting therapy is not recommended without proper study. Various scientific studies have proven the effects of fasting on chronic diseases, and I can, therefore, confidently recommend it as a therapy for beating and preventing many diseases.

What Does the Evidence Show?

We've discussed the different kinds of studies that were conducted to determine the effects of fasting on chronic disease; it's time we consider the results of these studies and how fasting has been proven to increase your overall well-being and beat and prevent chronic conditions.

Well, the results of the Longo and Mattson study (2014) yielded some very interesting results. They discovered that prolonged fasting is not only beneficial in many ways for combating cancer but it can also prevent cellular aging, which is one of the causes of several other chronic conditions, including dementia, arthritis, and osteoporosis. In the first part of their study, Longo and Mattson discussed the effects of prolonged fasting on cancer cells. They discovered that while regular (healthy) bodily cells enter a protected state during starvation, and the body focuses on repair (autophagy) and preservation, cancer cells do not have this ability.

Instead, they rely on constant nutrients to grow and survive. This resulted in healthy cells building a higher resistance to stress than cancer cells. The interesting part of this study is that healthy cells also developed a higher resistance to chemo toxicity while cancer cells, which were already weakened by the fasting protocol, were greatly affected by chemotherapy. This means that prolonged fasting can not only slow the growth of cancer cells but can also make chemotherapy more effective.

In addition, because the healthy cells are more resistant to stress, they are not as affected by chemotherapy. The studies done on mice concluded that prolonged fasting helped preserve bone marrow cells, which are crucial for a strong immune system. As such, prolonged fasting can help prevent the spread of cancer, increase chemotherapy's efficacy, and strengthen the immune system, which is linked to various other chronic conditions, especially autoimmune diseases.

Their studies also found that black hooded rats who experienced a prolonged fasting period of three days weekly for ten weeks did not experience hypoglycemia during a 2-hour strenuous swimming session compared to a control group that did not undergo prolonged fasting (Longo & Mattson, 2014). They attributed this to the fact that the rats that experienced prolonged fasting had larger glucose storages, as their bodies adapted to storing more glucose to use when fasting. This indicates that fasting could also help people with hypoglycemia or diabetes to store and regulate their blood glucose levels.

The Michalsen and Chenying (2013) study explained "Further beneficial effects of fasting are supported by observational data and abundant evidence from experimental research which found caloric restriction and intermittent fasting being associated with deceleration or prevention of most chronic degenerative and chronic inflammatory diseases." Their observations were based on the works of other researchers over many years. By reducing inflammation in the body, intermittent fasting can help prevent and beat inflammatory chronic conditions, such as IBS, Alzheimer's, and inflammatory heart disease.

As mentioned, many other studies have discovered the effects of prolonged fasting on several chronic diseases. Additionally, the research that discovered the impact of fasting on autophagy, increased HGH, and ketosis has also helped researchers explain many of the health benefits people who embrace prolonged fasting experience. While there is still a lot we can discover about prolonged fasting and its effect on chronic disease, the existing research is enough to convince thousands to at least consider it as a treatment option for their conditions. Many of these people have combated or beaten their chronic diseases and have embraced prolonged fasting as a regular part of their lives.

Human Studies for Fasting and Chronic Disease

You may have noticed that most of the research discussed above is based on the results of animal testing and observational studies. This might make you wonder why more human studies aren't conducted and if we can apply the effects witnessed during animal studies to humans. When it comes to human clinical studies, the regulations for these studies are much stricter, and strict guidelines have been put in place to determine how long a person may legally go without food during a clinical study. As such, the results of longer periods of prolonged fasting are limited, and many of the benefits discussed above have not been conclusively proven in a clinical study setting for humans.

This is where clinics like the Buchinger Wilhelmi clinics are an invaluable resource for learning about the effects of prolonged fasting on humans specifically. While the confidentiality of their patients is a top priority, members at the Buchinger Wilhelmi clinic have witnessed just how beneficial prolonged fasting can be for curing and managing various chronic conditions. Otto Buchinger himself was diagnosed with rheumatoid polyarthritis in 1917, which he eventually healed entirely with prolonged fasting. By carefully monitoring the health and progress of their patients, the Buchinger Wilhelmi clinic staff have been able to see first-hand how prolonged fasting affects humans and how it combats their chronic diseases.

Based on years of research and observation, the clinic is now able to prescribe a tailored prolonged fasting plan based on your chronic condition, which indicates that there is some variability in the effects of different fasting regimes and periods on different chronic diseases. Members of the clinic have also published some of their research and findings throughout the years, which serve as some scientific proof of the effects of fasting on humans. In addition to their studies, other research has also been published regarding the effects of prolonged fasting on people with chronic disease.

Despite the general lack of human studies for prolonged fasting, there is one well-recorded study of what is considered the longest fast in history. In 1965, Scot Angus Barbieri checked himself in at the *University Department of Medicine at the Royal Infirmary of Dundee* (Schuler, 2015). He reportedly stated that he was sick of being obese, weighing 456 lbs. at the time. He told the doctors that he was going to do prolonged fasting to lose some weight and improve his health, and the doctors were all too excited to monitor his progress. And they did—for 382 days! During this time, Angus was kept under constant medical supervision and given daily vitamins to ensure he didn't become deficient in any vitamins or minerals. After the fasting period, Angus weighed 180 lbs. and apart from going more than a month without a bowel movement, he didn't have any serious health complications.

Unfortunately, as Dr. Krista Varaday explained in *Men's Health* (Schuler, 2015), you wouldn't ethically be allowed to conduct or publish such research today, which is why this is such a unique study that displayed just how long the body can survive without food if it has enough stored fat to use for energy. Considering how strict ethics boards are these days, it's no surprise that there are very few prolonged fasting studies on humans to research. Fortunately, the studies conducted on animals, specifically mammals, give us a good indication of how people would react under the same circumstances. Much of the advice we are given today regarding fasting protocols is based on these animal studies.

The good news, however, is that people seem to have similar responses. And even though the research was not conducted on people, it has proven true for people as well. This means we can safely trust the results of these studies and implement the correct fasting protocols based on our specific chronic diseases.

The Future of Research in This Field

While human trials have been limited to date, the hope is that these recent animal trials will inspire other researchers to continue researching and monitoring the effects of prolonged and intermittent fasting on chronic disease. The effects of fasting on chronic disease may be well-established in previous studies, but that does not mean we know everything there is to know about fasting and chronic disease. On the contrary, there is still much we don't know and many ways we can improve in this field. What might future research focus on regarding fasting and chronic disease?

In addition to introducing more human studies for longer periods of fasting, future research may also help establish the best-prolonged fasting regimes for combating specific chronic diseases, such as cancer, heart disease, stroke, IBS, and more. By focusing on the effects of fasting on these diseases, researchers will be able to pinpoint exactly how long people should fast to see improvement and healing of these conditions. Research might also help determine the best fasting practices to eliminate or significantly reduce your chances of a specific chronic disease, especially if you have a higher risk of developing certain chronic conditions because of genetic and other factors.

Future research may also show us the best and safest ways of embracing prolonged fasting for specific conditions. And if all goes well, this research might be implemented in clinical trials for longer periods to really see how effective prolonged fasting is for combating chronic disease. Furthermore, the more research is conducted in the field of prolonged fasting and chronic disease, and the more people are made aware of the positive effects of fasting, the more influence this therapy will have in the scientific and medical community.

This means that more doctors and practitioners will start implementing and prescribing prolonged fasting as a treatment method for their chronically diseased patients. In time, more people will start implementing prolonged fasting in their regular lives, helping reduce the global chronic condition statistics, and reducing the risk of major chronic diseases, including cancer, heart disease, and diabetes, which are currently affecting millions of people worldwide. To think this is a free treatment option that could save millions of lives and reduce the burden on the medical system is awe-inspiring. Therefore, the hope is that influential researchers like Dr. Longo and others will continue to spread awareness of the effects of prolonged fasting and thereby help millions who believed they were doomed by their genetics or disease.

Key Takeaway From Chapter 8

There is plenty of scientific research backing the claims we have made in this book about the effects of prolonged fasting on chronic conditions. Prominent researchers, such as Dr. Valter Longo, the Buchinger Wilhelmi Clinic, and Dr. Eric Berg, have dedicated years of their lives to researching the effects and benefits of fasting in general. Dr. Valter Longo has intensively researched and studied the effects of prolonged fasting on cancer and various other chronic diseases, while the medical team at Buchinger Wilhelmi has been implementing these techniques in their clinics for four generations. Hopefully, the continued research will spread awareness about the effects of fasting on chronic conditions, helping to save the lives of millions of people living with these diseases.

Chapter 9:

Adopting an Anti-Chronic

Disease Fasting Lifestyle:

Actionable Steps

The previous chapters in this book focused on why prolonged fasting can improve chronic disease, which diseases it can improve, and what the science behind it all says about fasting and chronic disease. However, you might still not be too clear about implementing fasting into your lifestyle to achieve greater health and beat, prevent, and overcome chronic disease. That's what this chapter will focus on. This chapter will discuss actionable steps for implementing prolonged fasting into your lifestyle for improved health. Since this book primarily focuses on prolonged fasting, as it has been proven to deliver the greatest results for chronic disease, these actionable steps are all geared towards prolonged fasting.

In this chapter, you will learn some actionable steps for implementing prolonged fasting into your lifestyle in a safe and effective way. We'll share tips on how to prevent the side effects of prolonged fasting and the side effects that often accompany fast-breaking. We'll discuss biohacks that help enhance the effects of prolonged fasting. We'll also consider how you can combine prolonged fasting with other healthy lifestyle choices to reduce your risk of chronic disease and overcome it sooner. This is the chapter you have been waiting for—how to use prolonged fasting to beat and prevent chronic disease.

Building a Fasting Lifestyle—Your Actionable Steps

Now that you understand just how beneficial prolonged fasting may be for your health, especially if you are at risk for or currently suffer from a chronic disease. As previously mentioned, prolonged fasting is a more advanced or intense form of fasting. Therefore, we recommend getting familiar with fasting in general by trying some other fasting models, such as intermittent fasting first. You can use these actionable steps for intermittent fasting, too. And even though you may see enhanced benefits from prolonged fasting, you will still experience many health benefits from intermittent fasting. Once you have become more comfortable with fasting, you can try prolonged fasting. Here are some actionable steps you can implement when fasting to help manage your symptoms and make the experience more pleasant.

Step 1: Determine What You are Trying to Achieve

Before starting a new diet or lifestyle, you must determine what you are trying to achieve. Doing so can help you stay focused on your goals, particularly when you are hungry, moody, and want to quit. The same is true when fasting. Determining what you are trying to achieve before starting your fast, prolonged or intermittent, can increase your chances of success. For example, if your genetics increase your risk of breast cancer, you may wish to incorporate fasting in your lifestyle to reduce this risk and prevent you from getting cancer. If you have been warned about a risk for type-2 diabetes or heart disease because of your weight, you may wish to implement fasting for weight loss and to reduce your risk of diabetes.

As you know, there are many different fasting models, and your goals may determine which fasting model will work best for your needs. Of course, this means understanding the different fasting models and knowing which ones are best suited for different diseases. Therefore, you must do plenty of research before choosing a fasting model. Suppose your concerns are related to gut health, for example. In that case, if you suffer from chronic gastrointestinal disorder, leaky gut, or SIBO, you might consider reading the first book in this series to gain a better understanding of how fasting helps to improve those conditions.

Suppose you are concerned about your brain health, for example. In that case, if you are at greater risk for developing Alzheimer's, dementia, or depression, you may wish to read book two in this series to gain a greater understanding of how fasting affects brain health. Furthermore, suppose you have other specific concerns, such as cancer, heart disease, or IBS. In that case, you may consider researching the best fasting methods and practices for your specific health condition. The more informed you are, the better it is to make the right choices regarding fasting, food intake, and other practices.

How do you determine what you are trying to achieve? While there is usually one leading cause that draws people to fasting, such as a risk for chronic disease or an existing chronic illness, you likely want your fasting journey to accomplish various things, such as weight loss, improved digestive health, strengthened immunity, and more. These factors also affect your chosen fasting model and how you implement it. Therefore, the best way to determine which fasting model is right for you and your needs is to write down all your goals and research the best fasting methods for those goals.

As the saying goes, "Those who fail to plan; plan to fail." You want your first prolonged fasting experience to be a success. That means having everything planned and prepared before starting. Trust me, you don't want to wait until you have seething headaches before you head to the pharmacy for some electrolytes. Prolonged fasting is not something you should do on a whim. Instead, it takes planning and dedication. So, to give yourself the greatest chance of success, you must be prepared before you start. That includes having clear goals from your fasting experience and having everything you will need to make this experience a success in place.

There might never be a "perfect time" to try prolonged fasting. But I wouldn't recommend this fasting model when you are experiencing great amounts of stress at work or home. While fasting will relieve the effects of oxidative stress on your body, prolonged fasting is taxing, not only physically but also mentally and emotionally. Therefore, it is best to choose a less stressful time to try this fasting model. Alternatively, you can start with a fasting model that is easier on your body and will also help reduce the effects of oxidative stress, such as intermittent fasting. Determining what you want to achieve from your fasting experience can really help streamline the process and is a big determiner in the success or failure of your fasting journey.

Step 2: Prioritize Good Quality Food Intake

This is one point many people fail to grasp, and it leads to many failed fasting attempts and many horrible fasting side effects. Not to mention that it also affects the outcome of your fasting journey. The fasting lifestyle is about more than abstaining from food for predetermined periods. What you eat during your eating windows, before, and after concluding a fast is just as crucial as the fasting period itself. We've explained the value and importance of nutrition in Chapter 6. But now I would like to encourage you to prioritize good quality foods when eating.

For example, prolonged fasting is excellent for cancer prevention. But all those health benefits, such as cellular regeneration, autophagy, and increased resistance to stress, will all be for nothing if you fuel your body with cancer-causing foods in your eating window. What are cancer-causing foods? According to *Medical News Today* (Sherrell, 2023), the following foods may increase your risk of developing cancer:

- **Processed meats:** hot dogs, salami, sausages, bacon, corned beef, beef jerky, lunch meat, ham, spam, and more.

- **Processed foods:** soda, sugary cereals, packaged snacks including cookies and chips, modified spreads, fast food, sweets, candies, and more.

These foods all contain high amounts of preservatives, artificial ingredients, and sodium (not the good kind). They are linked to increasing your risk of cancer and may also cause various other chronic diseases, such as heart disease, diabetes, obesity, and IBS. Therefore, if you want to stay healthy and increase the efficiency of your fasting model, you should also focus on what you eat when not fasting. The best foods to eat are whole foods.

Whole foods are foods that have undergone minimal processing. The more farm-to-table you can eat, the better. In addition to whole foods, fasting experts, such as Dr. Berg (2018), also recommend including fermented foods, such as sauerkraut, kombucha, and kimchi, into your diet. Fermented foods are packed with micronutrients. They are also probiotics or prebiotics, which are crucial for optimal gut health and to assist the body's detoxification process. Fermented foods can also bring flavor and diversity to your diet, which can greatly help when your diet is restrictive due to calorie or other restrictions.

Of course, what you eat when breaking your fast is crucial, especially after a prolonged fast when your digestive system is more sensitive. When concluding a prolonged fast, you really want to ensure you feed your body the highest possible quality food. It doesn't have to be expensive or time-consuming to make. In fact, the simpler the food, the better. People often mistake good quality food intake for expensive groceries, but that's not the case.

Your food doesn't have to be organic or hand-reared. While these foods are higher in nutrients and contain fewer preservatives and pesticides, it isn't practical or economical for everyone to buy these types of foods. Instead, opt for the highest quality foods you can afford. If this means eggs, avocado, and seeds, then that's perfect! If you can afford organically grown produce, that is also great. If you can grow your own produce to use when cooking, even better! Focusing on whole foods packed with micronutrients, vitamins, and minerals will help your body recover from prolonged fasting (or any fasting) much better.

It will also ensure that all the hard work your body has put into cellular repair and regeneration gets put to good use. If you eat junk food and processed foods after fasting, you will undo all the positive effects of fasting on your body. But if you feed your body the right foods after fasting, it will use those foods to rebuild and replenish. As you already know, your first meal after breaking a prolonged fast is one of your most important meals. Opting for small, simple meals at this time will aid your digestion and help it wake up again and start producing the enzymes and chemicals needed for proper digestion.

Bone broth, vegetable soup, a cooked egg, or half an avocado are great examples of foods to conclude a prolonged fast with. Furthermore, suppose you want to ensure that you are fueling your body with the best foods you can. In that case, I recommend seeing a nutritionist who specializes in fasting to help you eat the right foods for your chronic condition and fasting model. Of course, drinking enough water; about half a gallon (2 liters) a day; and electrolytes is also crucial for your health and well-being. This not only applies to when you are fasting but to when you are eating as well.

Step 3: Choose Your Fast (It Can Be More Than One Type)

This book has mainly focused on prolonged fasting. However, we also shared various other fasting models, including intermittent fasting (alternate-day fasting, time-restricted eating, and more), water fasting, dry fasting, and fast mimicking. While prolonged fasting certainly has the most proven benefits for chronic disease, it is not the only fasting model that will deliver results. Prolonged fasting is not for everyone, and it might not be for you. As a matter of fact, as we have discussed previously, it is not recommended that you jump straight into prolonged fasting.

Instead, based on your research and knowledge of different fasting models, you may choose another fasting model to begin with. Starting with an easier fasting model is not a sign of weakness. In fact, it may improve your chances of success. Even if you start with a 12/12 fasting protocol, which means you are only fasting for around four hours a day (if you sleep the other 8 hours of your fasting time), you will still experience some benefits from fasting. As you become more comfortable with fasting and don't feel as hungry anymore while fasting, you can gradually increase your fasting periods until you reach your desired fasting model.

Fasting is a lifestyle, not a diet. This means that fasting needs to be sustainable. Suppose your fasting model is so restrictive that you can no longer enjoy spending time with family or friends because of it, or you feel like you are becoming an unpleasant person to be around because you are always moody because you are fasting. In that case, it might be time to reconsider your current fasting model. You don't have to be on the same fasting model forever. Not even experienced fasters stay on the same fasting model indefinitely. In fact, there are certain circumstances in which fasting is not recommended at all.

If you are sick (not chronic conditions, but acute ones), recovering from immediate surgery, pregnant, or breastfeeding, then it might not be the best time to start a new fasting model. Ideally, you want your body to be as healthy and strong as possible when starting a fasting model to improve your chance of success and reduce the side effects you may experience during the fast. Of course, some people start fasting because they are sick or have chronic diseases, and that's another story. In this case, you should consult your primary physician before starting a new fasting model.

Certain conditions require medicine that must be taken with food. In this case, fasting might not be a suitable therapeutic option for you. You must recognize your limitations when choosing a fasting protocol. It's also important that you consider your situation at home. For example, if you have small children and you usually eat together as a family, it might cause upset or confusion if you suddenly stop eating with your loved ones. If you live with a person with a history of disordered eating, you might also reconsider fasting as they may find it triggering. Again, fasting is a lifestyle, and it therefore needs to be practical.

That being said, it's also important that you give yourself enough time to try a new fasting method before determining if it works or not. Your health will likely not change overnight, and there is bound to be an adjustment period when implementing fasting into your lifestyle, as there is with anything new. Therefore, it is recommended that you try a fasting model for at least three months before moving on to a new one or increasing your fasting period. This will give your body enough time to adjust to the fasting model. It will also give you enough time to adjust to the fasting model and to see if it can work in your current circumstances.

Taking notes during the fasting process can help you determine if the fasting model works for you. Instead of relying on how you feel or how much your health has improved, you will have more solid data to work with. We'll discuss monitoring your progress in greater detail in another section. If you have given the fasting model enough time to do its thing, and you still feel that it is not suitable for your lifestyle, then you can consider opting for another fasting model instead. The same is true if you want to increase your fasting time to yield greater results or if you don't feel like the fasting model is working well enough.

Step 4: Choose Your Eating Style

In addition to choosing your fasting model, you should also consider which eating style you want to follow. While you may choose to stick with your normal eating routine when not fasting, there are some eating styles that may yield better results when paired with fasting. Some of these models may also be better suited to your lifestyle or may prove more beneficial for certain chronic conditions. Here are some eating styles you could potentially choose from if you want to add more changes to your diet in addition to introducing a fasting model.

The Ketogenic Diet

We've discussed ketosis quite a bit in this book, so it makes sense that it is included here. Many people combine fasting with a ketogenic diet to keep their bodies in ketosis even when they are not fasting. A ketogenic diet focuses on fat as the primary food source, followed by proteins, dairy, and finally, carbs. Very little carbs and sugars are consumed as they will interrupt the ketogenic process. There are various health benefits of the ketogenic diet, and it may prove valuable to people who want to lose weight, prevent diabetes, or prevent heart disease while fasting.

Low-Sugar Diet

A low-sugar diet may be similar to a ketogenic diet, or it may involve cutting out all artificial and natural sugars. This diet may focus on lean meats, healthy fats, vegetables, and low-sugar fruits, such as berries. Starchy vegetables, such as potatoes, sweet potato, and corn, will likely be limited on a low-sugar diet as these foods are converted to sugar by the body and will cause blood glucose spikes. A low-sugar diet is often recommended for people at risk of developing diabetes or heart disease. It is also recommended for obese people as they are at greater risk for these conditions. A low-sugar diet may also result in ketosis in the body, especially if it focuses on healthy fast as the primary energy source.

Whole Foods Diet

A whole food diet involves eating only fresh, whole foods, such as fresh fruits and vegetables, fresh meat, and (sometimes) raw dairy. Depending on how strict you are on the whole food diet, you may purchase cheese and processed dairy products. However, processed meats, fast foods, and other processed foods and snacks are not permitted on this diet. People on whole foods diet often process their own foods to bake bread and pastries. Following a whole foods diet gives you more control over what you put in your body. It also reduces the number of preservatives, pesticides, and chemicals you consume, which can help prevent and beat many chronic conditions, including cancer and inflammatory conditions.

Vegetarian/Vegan Diet

Some people prefer a vegetarian/vegan diet in addition to prolonged fasting. A vegetarian diet may prove useful if you have difficulty digesting meats. While the scientific evidence for the health benefits of a vegetarian or vegan diet for improved chronic disease is contradictory and somewhat lacking in substance, it may be worth a try if you find that your chronic disease flares up when consuming large amounts of meat or animal products. Of course, if your reasons for going vegetarian or vegan are religious or ethical, then you are free to do so as well. But be aware that a vegetarian or vegan diet does not automatically mean healthy. Many vegetarian meat substitutes have as many preservatives and chemicals as processed meats.

Whether you implement a new eating style into your diet in addition to fasting or not is your choice. I would, however, recommend doing so in phases. Choosing a strict diet, such as a ketogenic diet, and then starting a 16/8 intermittent fasting protocol at the same time might be overwhelming and will reduce your chances of success. It's also important to discuss new diets with your physician if you already have a chronic disease, as certain diets may be counterproductive to your medication or treatment. Furthermore, you should ensure that you are consuming enough calories in your eating window to prevent malnourishment and the side effects that come with it.

Just like the different fasting models, you can also experiment with different eating styles to see which ones work best for you and have the greatest benefits for your chronic disease. It's also important that you give each new diet at least 8–12 weeks before determining if it is beneficial or not. And, of course, it's important to drink enough water, get good quality sleep, and focus on healthy habits in general to give your eating plan the best chance of success. Monitoring your progress and mood can help you determine if your current eating plan and fasting model are working or if you need to make some adjustments.

Step 5: Measure Your Progress

If you want to be successful in your fasting journey, you need a measure to determine how you are progressing. This is why measuring your progress is important. How you measure your progress depends on various factors, such as your goals with fasting, the eating plan you incorporate, the fasting model you have chosen, and your overall health before fasting. The type of chronic disease you are trying to combat will also affect how you monitor your progress. Some chronic diseases are easier to monitor than others. For example, if your goal is weight loss for diabetes prevention, you will know your current plan works if you lose weight.

But if your goal is cancer or stroke prevention, you will likely never know if your plan is working—the absence of the disease will be your primary indicator. Other chronic diseases require blood tests to determine if your fasting plan is working. But if there is no definitive way to tell if your plan is working, you may feel that it is not. You may become discouraged and eventually quit your new fasting lifestyle despite any invisible progress you have made. Therefore, it's important to consider how you can monitor your progress aside from tracking your chronic disease progression.

This is where practical, short-term goals come into play. Considering how many health benefits there are of fasting, beating chronic disease may not be your only goal. Let's take oxidative stress as an example. Oxidative stress wreaks havoc on your body. It puts strain on your immune system, affects your digestive system, and has a significant impact on your mental health. It also increases your risk of stroke, which is why many people focus on reducing the effects of oxidative stress. Oxidative stress occurs due to by-products of oxygen metabolism but can also be increased by other factors, such as pollution, heavy metals, and preservatives (Pizzino et al., 2017).

Considering how much damage oxidative stress can cause, fasting is one of the methods often employed when combating it. Since fasting increases autophagy, it can effectively cleanse the cells from oxidative stress, reducing its effects on your body. But how can you tell if your fasting plan is working for reducing oxidative stress and preventing stroke? One way of measuring the success of your fasting plan is by measuring your sleep progress and mental health. Oxidative stress increases anxiety. So, if you feel less anxious or experience fewer panic attacks, notice an increase in your sleep patterns, and feel more energized overall, it is a sign that your fasting lifestyle effectively reduces oxidative stress.

This is one example of how you can monitor your progress. Overall, a fasting model and eating plan will improve your overall health. If you notice improvements in your energy levels, the health of your skin and hair, improvements in your mood, weight loss, and a general greater sense of health, you can rest assured that your fasting plan is working. Of course, you may experience some ups and downs in your health when you first start a new fasting plan, especially as your body adjusts to your new lifestyle and enters a purging phase. In a purging phase, your body enters a detox overdrive and expels many toxins and pollutants at once. People often experience symptoms such as headaches, skin breakouts, and fatigue at this time.

This is why it is important to give your fasting plan a few months to work before you judge its effectiveness. You may start experiencing improvements within a few weeks, but you won't experience the full range of benefits immediately. Giving your fasting plan at least 12 weeks will help you determine how effective it is and where you can make adjustments to make it even more effective. Furthermore, by keeping a journal or measuring your progress with statistical data (sleep tracking, weight monitoring, ketone levels, and more), you can get a clear image of how well your plan is working.

Remember that there will be highs and lows during your fasting period. This is not a short-term weight loss hack; this is a lifestyle change—one your future self will thank you for. So, finding things to distract yourself when you feel hungry or want to quit during a prolonged fast can help you focus on what is really important and will improve your chances of success. If you feel like your current fasting plan is not working after 12 weeks, you may consider how to adjust it for greater success and improved health. You shouldn't feel ashamed if you have to step away from fasting for a while, and remember that you are on your own journey—it's okay if it does not look the same as everyone else's.

Step 6: Live in a Safe Environment

While you can do everything in your power to improve your health and reduce your risk of chronic disease, your results will be limited if your environment is not conducive to healthy living. There are a couple of different factors to consider if you want to live in a healthy environment and increase your chances of success. Not only can these factors affect the results of your fasting and diet, but they might actually increase your risk of chronic disease. So, let's consider the factors that may affect your fasting journey and how you can ensure that you live in a safe environment that encourages healing and healthy living.

Remove Mold From Your House

If you live in a high-humidity area, you may experience mold growth in certain parts of your home, such as closets, around windows, and in the attic. Mold also frequently grows in the bathroom, where there tends to be more moisture. And while you may think that a bit of mold is harmless, it is not. Mold can lead to allergies, sinus infections, and Aspergillosis. It can also affect your melatonin production, which results in poor sleep quality. This can interfere with the effects of your fasting plan and may lead to poor health. Therefore, it's important to remove mold from your house with a mold killer. Ensure the area is well-ventilated after use so you don't breathe those chemicals in.

Avoid Heavy Metals

Heavy metals, such as lead, mercury, arsenic, thallium, and cadmium, are often found around your house. They are found in household items, such as ceramic crockery, non-stick pots and pans, water, food, rugs, and other daily items. These metals are ingested in microscopic amounts when you use items that contain them or eat food tainted with them, and they can lead to severe health complications, including diarrhea, a prickly sensation in your hands and feet, weakness, dehydration, and abdominal pain. They will also interfere with your hormones and general health, which could lead to chronic disease. Removing all traces of heavy metals in your house can be nearly impossible.

Therefore, a heavy metal detox diet is recommended to detox your body from the heavy metals it has absorbed. This diet includes avoiding metal-containing foods, such as fish, alcohol, and brown rice, and eating foods, such as cilantro, curry, probiotics, tomatoes, green tea, and garlic, to detoxify your body and reduce the effects of heavy metals.

Steer Clear From Ammonium Nitrate Fertilizers

Ammonium nitrate fertilizers are commonly used to fertilize grass and garden beds around the house. And while its use outside is perfectly safe, it can cause skin irritation and airway infections if it is inhaled. Therefore, it's important to keep your fertilizers and other chemicals away from your home. Store them in a well-ventilated shed and only enter it if needed. A shower may be advisable after using some of these chemicals, as they can absorb through the skin and cause health complications.

Reduce Plastic Usage

Plastic products are all around us. They are cheap, convenient, and lightweight. But they also contain formaldehyde and melamine. Formaldehyde is a known carcinogen, while melamine is known to leach chemicals when exposed to heat. Therefore, if you use a plastic bowl in the microwave or pour hot substances into it, you may expose your food and your body to formaldehyde. Therefore, it is better to use glass or stainless steel takeaway mugs and only heat your food in glass containers to reduce exposure to toxic chemicals leaching into your food.

Limit Air Fryer Use

Air fryers have taken over our kitchens and our cooking practices. While they are a healthier alternative to deep-frying, and take less time than oven-cooking, the process of air frying may release a carcinogen known as acrylamide. Therefore, if you enjoy using your air fryer, it is recommended that you cook your food in a lower setting to reduce the amount of acrylamide exposure. Furthermore, opting for occasional air fryer use instead of frequent one can also reduce your exposure to this chemical and may help prevent cancer.

Consider an Air Purifier

If you live in an area with poor air quality, you may be exposed to pollutants from outside. The pollutants can cause health conditions and chronic disease. Furthermore, you may also suffer from allergies if you are constantly exposed to pollen and debris from outside that enters your home through the air. In this case, an air purifier, specifically one with a HEPA filter, can help improve the air quality inside your home. This can help your body fight off infection, improve your immune system, and prevent chronic disease. If you constantly struggle with airway infections or allergies, you may consider investing in an air purifier.

Step 7: Accompany Fasting With Biohacks

According to *Medical News Today,* "Biohacking is a term used to describe do-it-yourself biology. It involves people making incremental changes to their bodies, diet, and lifestyle to improve their health and well-being" (Geng, 2022). There are many different biohacks, some of which are entirely safe to try at home; others, not so much. But incorporating some of the safe biohacks into your fasting lifestyle can help reduce the fasting side effects you experience and may lead to enhanced results and greater health. Fasting is also a biohack used by many worldwide for improved health. Let's consider some biohacks that may prove beneficial if you want to improve your health and prevent chronic disease.

Sun Exposure

Did you know that 15 minutes of sunlight a day can significantly improve your mood, reduce anxiety, and manage depression? Sun exposure is a crucial thing for any living organism. Reptiles bathe in the sun, flowers turn to face the sun, and even nocturnal animals require some sun exposure for optimal health. Sunlight is a great source of vitamin D. Unfortunately, most of us spend all our time indoors and rarely get outside to feel the sun on our faces. Making a point of getting more exposure to sunlight can improve your health and well-being and might also prevent chronic conditions. Just remember to wear sunscreen!

Exercise

Exercise, or moving your body, also has many health benefits. It is not only good for weight loss and increased bone density, but it also regulates your mood and increases dopamine production, which can combat depression and anxiety. Exercise is also physically taxing, which can help you sleep better by making you tired. Incorporating 30 minutes of moderate exercise into your daily routine will significantly improve your mental and physical health and well-being. You can do whatever exercise you like, such as yoga, running, strength training, or simply walking outside.

High-Quality Sleep

People often neglect the importance of good-quality sleep for their overall health. Sleep reduces oxidative stress, calms the central nervous system, increases cellular regeneration, and improves your mood. It's an easy way to fast for longer, as you don't think about food when you are sleeping. To ensure you get high-quality sleep, avoid caffeine before bedtime, ensure your room is dark, quiet, and cool, and aim for at least seven hours of sleep daily. These factors impact the quality of your sleep. Once you start noticing improvements in your sleep, you will notice improvements in your health.

Meditation

Meditation is another helpful biohack that has been used by many cultures worldwide for thousands of years. Meditation improves your mind-body connection, soothes your central nervous system, improves your breathing, and promotes relaxation and healing. There are many different kinds of meditation to choose from, such as mindfulness meditation and movement meditation. Meditation can also be anything you find relaxing, such as journaling, taking a long bubble bath, or singing. Meditation is great for your mental and physical health. For a more detailed explanation of different fasting types, read Book 2 in this series: *Revitalize Your Brain After 40 With Fasting*.

Breathing Techniques

Like meditation, breathing techniques are a great way to soothe your central nervous system (which gets activated if you are stressed, anxious, or scared). An overactive central nervous system increases anxiety and leads to oxidative stress, which can compromise your immune system and digestive system. It may also increase your risk for chronic disease. Breathing techniques, such as box breathing (4 seconds in through the nose, 4 seconds hold, 4 seconds out through the mouth, 4 seconds hold, repeat), can soothe the central nervous system and reduce anxiety. Box breathing is a great way to increase oxygen intake and reduce heart rate.

Time in Nature

Spending more time in nature is another great way to improve your mental and physical health. Spending time in nature will increase your exposure to sunlight. It can soothe the central nervous system, reduce stress, and improve mood. When you are spending time in nature, it's also recommended that you walk barefoot, especially on grass. It reduces inflammation, improves your posture, regulates your heartbeat, and prevents insomnia (Bhardwaj, 2021). Spending time outside also increases your exposure to oxygen, helps your eyesight, and is a way to activate all your senses, creating harmony within your body.

Connecting With Loved Ones (or Pets)

Human beings are not meant to be solitary. Exposure to other humans and animals is crucial for mental and physical health. We know this by observing the health and behavior of people who have been void of interaction with others for some time, such as prison inmates punished with solitary confinement. Connecting with other people can significantly improve your mental and physical health. Studies have also shown that interaction with animals, such as dogs and cats, may have a similar effect (Hamblin, 2019). So, if you live alone or work from home, it might be time to adopt a fur baby.

Step 8: Exposure to Cold Shower

Cold exposure therapy, such as ice baths, is something we often see professional athletes do for improved recovery and increased performance. But cold exposure can help in many ways other than recovery. According to Dr. Susanna Søberg, cold therapy can improve your health right away—there is an acute response in the body when you enter the cold. Cold therapy can also improve your health in the long run by reducing the risk of lifestyle-related chronic disease. Furthermore, she explains that cold therapy can increase your health by enhancing your resistance to stress—both mentally and physically (Chatterjee, 2023).

Taking a cold shower can increase your metabolism, which helps to regulate blood sugar levels and promote weight loss. Interestingly enough, cold shower therapy can also change the microflora in your gut, which helps regulate how you digest food. Studies have shown that cold therapy can change gut flora to make it more effective at preventing diabetes (Lassila, 2021). Cold shower therapy is also a great recovery tool, as it can reduce lactic acid buildup in the muscles and reduce inflammation throughout the body, helping you recover faster after an intense workout. Reduced inflammation also has significant benefits for preventing and combating chronic disease.

"Cold stress has been proven to reduce the level of serotonin in most parts of the brain, which can help reduce exercise-related fatigue" (Lasilla, 2021). Therefore, cold shower therapy can reduce insomnia and improve sleep quality, which we have already determined is extremely important for your health and chronic disease prevention. Cold shower therapy also tricks the body into activating the sympathetic nervous system, and it then releases endorphins. Endorphins are known to improve your mood and combat depression and anxiety. Therefore, cold shower therapy may also reduce chronic mental conditions.

How can you incorporate cold shower therapy into your daily routine? An article published in UCLA Health says to keep the water below 60°F and to start slow. Try to stay in the cold water for about 30 seconds at the beginning, and gradually work your way up to 2 to 3 minutes of cold shower exposure. You can do this therapy daily or however, frequently you are comfortable with. Incorporating cold shower therapy into your lifestyle will enhance the effects of your fasting regime and may deliver some additional results as well.

If you want to take things up a notch, you can alternate between cold and hot water. Contrast heat therapy has many health benefits and can condition your body to get used to different environments. It may also make your cells more resistant to stress, which is beneficial when undergoing chemotherapy. However, contrast heat therapy is not a pleasant experience and is often left to professional athletes who really want to improve their recovery and performance. If you are interested in trying contrast heat therapy, it is recommended that you discuss it with your doctor first, especially if you have a heart condition.

To do contrast heat therapy, you will take a hot shower for 3 minutes. The water should not be scorching hot; it should be a comfortable temperature instead. Switch to a cold shower immediately after the hot one for 1 minute. Repeat this process three times, ending with the cold shower. You may experience skin sensitivity during this process as the nerve endings in your skin become more sensitive to temperature changes. You can incorporate contrast temperature therapy once a week or however, frequently you are comfortable with it.

Cold shower therapy is one biohack that has been used by many around the world. People used to be more exposed to the elements than we are today, so they usually experienced a natural form of temperature therapy when going about their day-to-day lives. However, now that we have indoor heating, air conditioners, and clothes made from various materials to keep us comfortable, we are no longer used to experiencing cold temperatures.

Step 9: Use Biohack Tools if Possible

Biohack tools are tools that you can use to make biohacking easier. There are many biohack tools available. Some are affordable and easy to use, while others are a bit more expensive and complex. You don't have to use biohack tools if you don't want to. However, they can make your new fasting lifestyle a bit easier to manage. Consider some biohack tools you can introduce into your lifestyle for improved health and well-being. We'll divide this section into two. The first part will be affordable biohacking tools you can use at home. The second part will give you an idea of some of the more advanced biohacking tools on the market that can improve your health even further.

Affordable and Home-Friendly Biohacking Tools

You may already have some of these tools. Biohacking tools include anything that increases your quality of life and is based on "biological principles." For example, they can improve your health and help you track your progress while fasting or introduce a new lifestyle plan for improved health and chronic disease prevention. Some of the best affordable biohacking tools include:

- **Smartwatches and fitness watches:** These devices can be used to monitor your progress and movement throughout the day. They can track how many steps you have walked, your average heart rate and breathing, and your activity level. These statistics are great to have on hand when tracking your progress, especially if you want to increase your activity level or reduce your stress (they track stress by monitoring your heart rate).

- **Blue light filtering glasses:** If you spend a lot of time in front of the computer, your eyes are exposed to blue light for long periods. Blue light is known to interrupt your sleeping patterns and may result in insomnia, poor sleep, and blurry vision. Anti-blue light glasses are affordable and can reduce the effects of blue light on your eyes and body.

- **White noise machine:** A white noise machine can improve sleep quality by targeting certain brain waves. This helps calm your mind and body. In addition to improving sleep quality, white noise can reduce stress and soothe your central nervous system. If you don't have a white noise machine, you can search for white noise music online or on your music streaming device.

Advanced Biohacking Tools

If you want to experiment with biohacking tools, you can also try some more advanced tools. These are generally more expensive, and you often must visit a clinic or special location to access these tools. If you have a specific problem and think these tools may offer a solution, they are well worth trying. However, if you do not have the means to use them, or if they are not available in your area, you can find other ways to try and achieve the same results. Here are some advanced biohacking tools you may consider using:

- **Hyperbaric oxygen chamber:** These chambers are airtight and supply you with 100% oxygen inside the chamber. Hyperbaric oxygen chambers are primarily used in hospitals to treat open wounds, but they can be used in a therapeutic setting as well. Hyperbaric oxygen chambers offer many health benefits, including advanced wound healing and reduced inflammation.

- **Sensory deprivation chamber:** The chambers are filled with salty water. If you get in them, you will be deprived of all your senses. The chambers are pitch black, quiet (and soundproof). The water is body temperature, so you don't feel it, and its salt concentration allows you to float in the water. Sensory deprivation chambers can soothe the sympathetic nervous system, reduce anxiety, and improve overall health.

- **Joovv light:** A Joovv light is a special light that combines red light and near-infrared light technology for improved healing. The different settings on this light provide different healing benefits, such as skin healing, reduced inflammation, enhanced recovery, strengthened immunity, and increased cellular regeneration.

These are merely some of the biohacking tools available. They may provide you with enhanced results from your fasting and lifestyle changes. Consult with your primary healthcare practitioner before trying any of these biohacking tools, especially if you are already undergoing treatment for a chronic disease.

Step 10: Vary Your Fast

Another thing to keep in mind is that your fasting regime may change as your health goals and needs change. For example, if you are fasting for weight loss now, you may choose to focus on another area of your health when you have reached your goal weight. In that case, another fasting model may better suit your needs. Or, if you are used to having a strict routine that allows for a strict fasting method, but you then go on holiday, and your routine is thrown out the window, then you might require a more flexible fasting model that you can adjust according to the daily changes.

In addition, if you have a child or even adopt a new pet, your responsibilities might make your current fasting model impractical. As mentioned before, fasting is a lifestyle, not a fixed-term diet. And for a lifestyle to be sustainable, it must be flexible. So, if you notice that your current fasting model no longer allows you to live your life to the fullest, it might be time to consider a new fasting model. Also, as your goals change, so too will your fasting model. For example, if you are focused on overall health and then get diagnosed with a chronic disease, you may rethink your fasting model to tailor it to fight your chronic disease.

Of course, you may also wish to increase your fasting time if you are building up to a specific time-restricted fasting model or even to a prolonged fasting model. In this case, you will frequently change your fasting routine to keep it aligned with your goals. There is absolutely nothing wrong with varying your fast, and there is no evidence to suggest that it may harm your health. However, there are certain things to remember when changing your fasting model or making other lifestyle changes as your goals change.

You may Experience Fasting Side Effects

Just because your body is used to fasting to some extent, it doesn't mean there won't be a transition period when you change to a new fasting model. Be prepared to experience some fasting side effects when changing your fasting model or the length of your fasting periods. These side effects may be less severe than those you experienced during your first fasting experience. You may also experience new side effects that you have not dealt with before. It is all a normal part of your body adjusting to the new fasting model.

Monitor Your Progress

When you change your fasting lifestyle, you must continue to monitor your progress. You can use the same techniques we discussed above. Monitoring your progress can help you determine if your new fasting model is working as well as the previous one, better or worse. Of course, you should first give your body some time to adjust to the new fasting regime, but once it has, you can start comparing the different fasting models you have tried to determine which ones work best for your health and which are most effective for combating your chronic condition.

Stick to the Fasting Model for 12 Weeks

As with your first fasting experience, you must give a new fasting model at least 8–12 weeks before determining if it works for you or not. There will always be some adjustment period to account for. If you want to give the new fasting model the best chance of success (or failure), you need to give it some time to start working before you judge it as better or worse. Monitor your chronic condition during this time to see how the new fasting model improves or aggravates it.

Don't Make Significant Changes

While adjusting your fasting model or fasting length is fine, you don't want to make too many changes at once. This will make it difficult to determine which parts of the fasting model are effective and which changes are unnecessary or harmful. Therefore, it is recommended that you only change one element of your fasting regime at a time—either the duration of the fast or the frequency at which you fast. This will also allow you to monitor your body's reaction to each change better, giving you a better idea of which fasting aspects you respond well to.

Listen to Your Body

While you should certainly monitor your progress and health during a fasting period, you must also listen to your body. If you are experiencing severe side effects from a new fasting model, your chronic disease has flared up, and you just feel horrible during the entire experience, it could be your body's way of saying that this is not a beneficial fasting model. In that case, you can revert back to the previous model or suspend fasting altogether for a while as you determine the exact cause of your side effects.

Below you will find a table with a summary of how you can incorporate these actionable steps into your lifestyle successfully.

YOUR ACTIONABLE STEPS
(A Summary)

Step 1: Determine what you want to achieve

It helps you

- Focus on your goals
- Increase your chances for success
- Determine your ideal fasting model

You need to

- Plan and prepare everything before starting your fasting journey
- Write down all your goals and do plenty of research before choosing a fasting model to understand which ones are suited for your disease
- Choose a less stressful time to try this fasting model
- Start with a fasting, e.g., IF model that is easier on your body to reduce the effects of oxidative stress

Example

If your genetics increase your risk of breast cancer, your fasting lifestyle should seek to reduce this risk and prevent you from getting cancer

Step 2: Prioritize good quality food intake

Important

- What you eat during your eating windows, before, and after breaking a fast is just as crucial as the fasting period itself

- If you eat junk and processed foods after fasting, you will undo all the positive effects of fasting on your body
- If you feed your body the right foods after fasting, it will use those foods to rebuild and replenish
- Probiotics or prebiotics, are crucial for optimal gut health and assist the body's detoxification process
- Avoid cancer-causing foods in your eating window such as, processed meats and foods
- The highest possible quality food doesn't have to be expensive. The simpler the food, the better
- Opt for the highest quality foods you can afford, organically produced or not, such as eggs, avocado, and seeds

You should

- Prefer whole or farm-to-table foods that have undergone minimal processing
- Choose probiotics, prebiotics, and fermented foods, such as sauerkraut, kombucha, and kimchi.
- Have bone broth, vegetable soup, a cooked egg, or half an avocado to conclude a prolonged fast
- Hydrate well and have enough electrolyte drinks

Step 3: Choose your fast

Important tips

- Choosing your fast carefully, based on your research and knowledge increases your chances of success.
- Fasting is a lifestyle, not a diet, and it needs to be practical and sustainable
- You must recognize your limitations when choosing a fasting protocol
- Give yourself enough time to try a new fasting method before determining if it works or not (8-12 weeks)
- You can start with a 12/12 fasting protocol, fast for around four hours a day. Become more comfortable with fasting and gradually increase your fasting periods until you reach your desired fasting model
- Taking notes during the fasting process can help you determine if a fasting model works for you

Examples of fasting models you can try

- Intermittent fasting (alternate-day fasting, time-restricted eating, and more)
- Water fasting
- Dry fasting
- Fast mimicking
- Prolonged fasting

Step 4: Choose your eating style

Important

- Some eating styles may yield better results when paired with fasting. They may also be better suited to your lifestyle or may prove more beneficial for certain chronic conditions

- It's essential that you give each new diet at least 8-12 weeks before determining if it is beneficial or not
- Many vegetarian meat substitutes have as many preservatives and chemicals as processed meats
- I would recommend that you implement a new eating style into your diet in addition to fasting in phases

You can combine

- Fasting with a ketogenic diet to keep your bodies in ketosis even when you are not fasting
- Fasting with low sugar diet involves cutting out all artificial and natural sugars. And focus on lean meats, healthy fats, vegetables, and low-sugar fruits, such as berries, and low consumption of starchy vegetables
- A whole food diet with fasting involves eating only fresh, whole foods, such as fresh fruits and vegetables, fresh meat, and (sometimes) raw dairy
- Vegetarian/vegan with fasting. However, be aware that a vegetarian or vegan diet does not automatically mean healthy

Step 5: Measure your progress

Important tips

- Have practical, short-term goals toward your ultimate goal. e.g., you can focus on reducing the effects of oxidative stress knowing your end goal is to decrease the risks of stroke and heart diseases

- How you measure your progress depends on various factors such as, your goals, eating plan, the fasting model you have chosen, your overall health before fasting, and the type of chronic disease you are trying to combat

For example

- If your goal is weight loss for diabetes prevention, you will know your current plan works if you lose weight
- If you feel less anxious or experience fewer panic attacks, notice an increase in your sleep patterns, and feel more energized overall, it is a sign that your fasting lifestyle effectively reduces oxidative stress
- If you notice improvements in your energy levels, your mood, the health of your skin and hair, weight loss, and a general greater sense of health, you can rest assured that your fasting plan is working

Step 6: Live in a safe environment

Important

- Your results will be limited if your environment is not conducive to healthy living
- An unsafe environment might increase your risk of chronic disease

Actions you can take

- Remove mold from your house. Mold can lead to allergies, sinus infections, and Aspergillosis.

It can affect your melatonin production, which results in poor sleep quality.

- Avoid heavy metals. They can interfere with your hormones and general health, which could lead to chronic disease
- Steer clear from ammonium nitrate fertilizers. Its use outside is perfectly safe. However, it can cause skin irritation and airway infections if inhaled
- Reduce plastic usage. They contain formaldehyde and melamine. Formaldehyde is a known carcinogen, while melamine is known to leach chemicals when exposed to heat
- Limit air fryer use. The process of air frying may release a carcinogen known as acrylamide. It is recommended that you cook your food in a lower setting to reduce the amount of acrylamide exposure.
- Consider air purifier. This can help your body fight off infection, improve your immune system, and prevent chronic disease

For example

It is better to use glass or stainless steel takeaway mugs and only heat your food in glass containers to reduce exposure to toxic chemicals leaching into your food.

Step 7: Accompany fasting with biohacks

You can

- Make incremental changes to your body, diet, and lifestyle to improve your health and well-being

- Reduce the fasting side effects

A few biohacks
- Sun exposure. 15 minutes of sunlight a day can significantly improve your mood, reduce anxiety, and manage depression
- Exercise. Incorporating 30 minutes of moderate exercise into your daily routine will significantly improve your mental and physical health and well-being
- High-quality sleep. Sleep reduces oxidative stress, calms the central nervous system, increases cellular regeneration, and improves mood
- Meditation. Meditation improves your mind-body connection, soothes your central nervous system, improves your breathing, and promotes relaxation and healing
- Breathing techniques. Breathing techniques are a great way to soothe your central nervous system
- Time in nature. It can soothe the central nervous system, reduce stress, and improve mood
- Connecting with loved ones (or pets). Connecting with other people can significantly improve your mental and physical health

Important tips
- It's recommended that you walk barefoot, especially on grass, when spending time in nature. It reduces inflammation, improves your posture, regulates your heartbeat, and prevents insomnia

- The box breathing technique (4 seconds in through the nose, 4 seconds hold, 4 seconds out through the mouth, 4 seconds hold, repeat) is a great way to increase oxygen intake and reduce heart rate and anxiety

Step 8: Exposure to cold shower

Usefulness

- Reduces the risk of lifestyle-related chronic diseases
- Enhance resistance to stress
- Increase your metabolism
- Improves microflora in your gut
- Promote diabetes prevention
- Reduces inflammation
- Improves sleep quality
- Reduces chronic mental conditions

How to incorporate

- Start slow and keep the water below 60°F. Try to stay in the cold water for about 30 seconds at the beginning, and gradually work your way up to 2 to 3 minutes of cold shower exposure. Do this therapy daily or as frequently as you are comfortable with.

Important tips

- Contrast heat therapy (alternate between cold and hot water) makes your cells more resistant to stress
- Contrast heat therapy is beneficial when undergoing chemotherapy (however, discuss with the doctor first)

Step 9: Use biohacks tools if possible

Usefulness

- biohack tools make biohacking easier

Example

- smartwatches and fitness watches
- blue light filtering glasses
- white noise machine
- hyperbaric oxygen chamber
- sensory deprivation chambers
- Joovv light

Important tips

- A white noise machine can improve sleep quality by targeting certain brain waves. This helps calm your mind and body
- Smartwatches and fitness watches can track how many steps you have walked, your average heart rate and breathing, and your activity level

Step 10: Vary your fast

Important

- Very useful to suit your circumstance and meet specific needs
- You may experience fasting side effects
- You should
- Monitor your progress
- Stick to the fasting model of 12 weeks
- Not make significant changes
- Listen to your body

- Be prepared to experience some fasting side effects when changing your fasting model or the length of your fasting periods
- Monitor your progress to help you determine if your new fasting model is working as well as the previous one, better or worse

Key Takeaway From Chapter 9

There are many actionable steps you can take to increase your chances of success and make your fasting journey a much more pleasant experience. Determining what you wish to achieve from the fasting model can improve your focus and help you choose the right fasting model. Good quality food is crucial for improved health, especially before and after a prolonged fast. Prolonged fasting is but one fasting model; it is up to you to choose which one you think will work best. There are also various eating styles you can choose from to support your healthy lifestyle. Of course, you can also use biohacks and biohack tools to improve health and enhance the effectiveness of your fasting lifestyle.

Chapter 10:

Case Studies

While we've already discussed some examples and studies to prove that prolonged fasting can heal chronic disease, there are more factors to consider. Since most of the studies and research focus on animal studies, you may wonder how we know the same applies to people. Well, this is where case studies and anecdotal evidence come into play. We have collected data from various people's stories about how they overcame and managed chronic disease through fasting. In this chapter, we will review some of those case studies to motivate you to embrace fasting as a treatment method for your own disease.

Case Study #1: The Story of Jean-Jacques Throchon

The first case study really is an inspiring story of how alternative therapies, such as prolonged fasting, can significantly reduce the progression of chronic disease and potentially even cure it. Jean-Jeacques Throchon is a pilot who has spent his life flying the skies and surfing the waves. Then, in 2003, he was diagnosed with kidney cancer, which resulted in the immediate removal of his left kidney. Nine years later, his cancer returned with a vengeance, and he had malignant lung tumors. After undergoing more surgeries to try and remove the tumors, Jean-Jeacques' odds were not looking too bright. He was diagnosed with stage 4 cancer and was given around three years to live.

But Throchon was determined to live far longer than three years. He took to the internet and studied all he could about alternative therapies for cancer treatment. This brought him across the works of Valter Longo and other fasting specialists. Jean-Jeacques took a keen interest in exploring how he could use fasting and other alternative therapies to conquer his cancer and take back his life. Fortunately, his research and dedication paid off! Throchon's oncologist was so impressed with the almost unbelievable turn in his diagnosis that he prompted Jean-Jeacques to record his journey so that others could learn from it too.

That's what Jean-Jeacques did. He released a book titled "Flying Against the Odds," where he shares a detailed explanation of his journey to overcome his cancer. He explains that he undertook a 12-day prolonged fast before the surgery on his lungs to remove the tumors. This resulted in half the tumors calcifying (dying) afterward because, as you know, cancer cells cannot survive the stress your body gets put under when fasting. Jean-Jeacques was adamant about sharing his journey and hopefully helping others realize the effectiveness of alternative therapies and fasting for overcoming cancer and other chronic diseases.

Case Study #2: Otto Buchinger's Tale

Dr. Otto Buchinger, as you already know, was the founder of the first Buchinger Wilhelmi Clinic. What you may not know, however, is that he started this clinic after prolonged fasting, which literally saved his life. During WWI, Buchinger served as a naval doctor. While he made a good name for himself, his plans were quickly overturned when he developed severe rheumatoid polyarthritis in 1917. His diagnosis was so poor, and his mobility so limited, that he was discharged from the navy as an invalid. As you can imagine, this severely affected Otto's mental and physical well-being.

At the time, Western medicine provided nearly no solution to his problem, and Otto was all but left to suffer and die from his disease. However, being a doctor himself, Buchinger continued to research possible cures. In 1919, Otto Buchinger started considering alternative therapies to cure rheumatoid polyarthritis. This led him to Dr. Riedlin in Freiburg, who recommended that he try prolonged fasting using traditional methods. Shortly after starting this prolonged fasting journey, Otto Buchinger's condition significantly improved, and several months later, he was entirely cured of the disease he thought would kill him.

After being cured of chronic disease with fasting, Otto Buchinger dedicated his life to researching and understanding prolonged fasting and its effects on the human body. He also focused on developing a medically sound fasting therapy that combined holistic medicine and also focused on emotional well-being. As a doctor and a spiritual person, Otto understood the importance of the spirit on the body and vice versa. And, as one can say, the rest is history. His research was so influential that it sparked three generations after him to continue his work and heal others with fasting therapy.

Case Study #3: How Fred Evrard Overcame Stage 3 Colon Cancer

Fred Evrard has been a health-conscious person since birth. He grew up in a martial arts family and practiced healthy eating habits for all his life. He never ate fast foods, smoked, drank soda, or and only ate organic food. Furthermore, he was a regular faster, practicing intermittent fasting and following a ketogenic diet. While he had a genetic risk for colon cancer (both his grandfather and father died of the disease), he assumed that his lifestyle had done enough to protect him against the effects of this disease. Since he led such an active, healthy lifestyle, Fred did not see the need to go for regular colonoscopies or have his risk for colon cancer assessed.

Unfortunately, colon cancer is one type of cancer that can be entirely genetic. This means that despite his best efforts, Fred still had an increased risk of developing colon cancer. And he did. After experiencing some cancer-related symptoms, such as bloody stool, psoriasis on his knees and elbows, and inflammation, for several months, Fred went to a doctor and was diagnosed with stage 3 colon cancer. As you can imagine, he was completely shocked by this diagnosis. At this time, he had a 4-inch tumor growing from his rectum to his colon, and was given a 50% chance of survival.

But this would include extensive chemotherapy, radiation therapy, and surgery. Knowing the effects of fasting and a ketogenic diet on cancer, Fred decided to try alternative therapies instead. He immediately started a 21-day prolonged fast, after which the tumor had shrunk by 50%. He followed that 21-day fast with intermittent fasting (one meal a day) and a strictly organic ketogenic diet. Within four months, Fred went from stage 3 colon cancer to remission. That shows how quickly your body can repair itself and rid itself of cancer cells if you follow the correct protocols.

Case Study #4: The Middle East Has the Lowest Cancer Statistics Worldwide

An interesting study has been published recently, and it has also been discussed by Dr. Eric Berg. This study considers why the Middle East (UAE, Yemen, Saudi Arabia, Qatar, Oman, and Kuwait) has the lowest cancer statistics worldwide. One of the reasons for this is that the Middle East is a primarily Islamic-dominant region. Part of the Islamic faith is Ramadan, an annual fasting period. Ramadan lasts one month, during which people fast from dusk until dawn. So, they are not even fasting for 30 days straight, and you can already see a tremendous decrease in their risk of developing cancer.

While Australians have a 468/100,000 chance of getting cancer, the highest country in the Middle East only has a 116/100,000 chance of getting cancer (Berg, 2021). This is a significant difference. But that's not the only reason why people in the Middle East have a reduced risk of cancer. Another reason is because of the spices they use.

Middle Eastern cuisine uses many spices for cooking. Some of these spices, such as coriander (cilantro), nutmeg, cinnamon, saffron, turmeric, carraway, and cardamom, have proven to reduce the risk of cancer and fight cancer cells.

Yet another reason why people in the Middle East have a lower risk of cancer is because alcohol is prohibited by the Islamic faith. Therefore, Muslims don't consume alcohol, a substance known to increase your risk of many chronic diseases, including liver and other cancers. Furthermore, women are not allowed to smoke or use tobacco products, further reducing their risk of tobacco-related cancers. This proves that intermittent fasting can improve the effectiveness of other factors that reduce your risk of cancer. While people in the Middle East still have other factors contributing to their cancer statistics, intermittent fasting is at least one reason they are not nearly as high as in many other countries.

Case Study #5: Fasting the Way Forward

Considering the discoveries we have made regarding the effects of prolonged fasting on your body and how well it affects your healthy cells and protects them against chemotherapy, scientists have started considering the potential health benefits of prolonged fasting for people who will travel to Mars in the future. The idea is that prolonged fasting will not only improve their general health and well-being while they endure the long-term travel to Mars, but it will also protect them against solar radiation. Solar radiation is a big concern for space travelers as they move out of the protective ozone layer around Earth and will come into closer contact with the sun.

One study published in the *National Library of Medicine* (Valayer et al., 2020) noted the following about the use of fasting to protect long-distance space travelers from radiation:

> "Caloric restriction and fasting have been shown to induce a variety of immediate and long-term physiological effects. The rapidly growing body of evidence of research that investigates the effects of caloric restriction and fasting indicates many benefits affecting numerous physiological systems" (p.1).

The idea that prolonged or intermittent fasting could protect space travelers against solar and ionizing radiation is fascinating. While research is ongoing to determine the exact fasting protocols that will be used during space travel, it is looking more and more like a viable option for space travelers to implement fasting in their nutritional protocols in space. Refer to the illustration at the end of this chapter for a visual depiction of this concept.

Case Study #6: The Rudolf Breuss Cancer Cure

Rudolf Breuss was an Austrian naturopath who developed what is now called Total Cancer Treatment. This treatment plan is very simple, affordable, and effective, according to the thousands of testimonies gathered in his book, very effective. Rudolf's cancer cure is based on the idea that cancer grows on proteins and solid food. Therefore, you can starve the cancer if you stop eating solid food. As we know from more recent research, there is some truth to this theory. Fasting sends the healthy cells into protective mode while starving the cancer cells. Rudolf Breuss' cancer cure involves a prolonged fast of 42 days.

During this time, you will consume water, herbal teas, and a specific vegetable juice blend consisting of beetroot, celery, potato, black radish, and carrots. According to Rudolf's theory, these vegetables contain all the nutrients the body needs to survive and thrive during the 42-day fast, while the cancer cells are starved of their nutrients. These vegetables contain plenty of antioxidants and nutrients that the body needs to stay healthy and naturally fight cancer. Furthermore, Breuss suggests several herbal tea blends, including kidney tea, to be taken at certain times during the fasting period.

While Rudolf Breuss' total cancer cure fast is certainly not for the faint of heart, it has thousands of grateful followers who have beaten their cancer by following this protocol. Furthermore, Breuss has many other fasting protocols for other chronic diseases and overall health. He also recommends certain herbal teas based on the type of cancer you have and prescribes when to take the teas and how much. While the reasoning behind his total cancer protocol is slightly outdated, the results speak for themselves, and it is a treatment plan to consider if you have been diagnosed with cancer.

Key Takeaway From Chapter 10

If you believe in the power of testimony, then you have now read plenty of case studies to convince you to try prolonged fasting to cure chronic disease. Jean-Jacques Throchon and Fred Evrard overcame their cancer with prolonged fasting, followed by intermittent fasting and other lifestyle changes. Otto Buchinger cured his rheumatoid polyarthritis with prolonged fasting and then dedicated his life to researching the effects of prolonged fasting. People in the Middle East have the lowest cancer statistics worldwide, partly because of their annual fast, and researchers are now considering prolonged fasting as a protection method against radiation for long-distance space travelers.

Fasting as a Potential Solution for Safer Human Spaceflight:

According to the European Space Agency (ESA), "A human expedition will one day set sail for Mars, but the dangerous radiation in interplanetary space is a major concern."

Fasting (IF and PF) could protect long-distance space travellers against solar and ionizing radiation.

More research is needed to determine the exact fasting protocol that will be used during space travel (Valayer et al., 2020).

Chapter 11:

Frequently Asked

Questions

Considering all the information you have learned throughout this book, you may still have some unanswered questions. Or perhaps there is some information you would like to be reminded of. Well, that's what this chapter is for. We will consider the top ten frequently asked questions about fasting and chronic disease to ensure you have all the information you need when starting your fasting journey. Most of these questions have been discussed in greater detail earlier in the book so that you can refer to previous chapters for a more detailed answer. So, let's consider the most frequently asked questions about prolonged fasting and chronic disease.

How Can I Overcome Constipation When I Fast?

Constipation is a common side effect of fasting. While your body will adjust to the lack of food and your constipation will improve, you may have some trouble with this when you first start fasting or during your first prolonged fast. If you are trying another fasting model, such as intermittent fasting, you can include more fiber in your diet in your eating window. Low GI carbs, like oats and fruits and vegetables, provide your body with plenty of fiber to help relieve constipation. Chia seeds mixed with water or milk to make a "chia pudding" can also improve your digestion.

During a prolonged fast, you might not be able to eat for a while. In this case, you can consider herbal teas with natural laxative properties, such as senna, chamomile, and licorice. Ensure you buy 100% herbal tea blends, not teas with added sugar or preservatives. Constipation may also arise if you are dehydrated. Therefore, ensuring you are properly hydrated and take enough electrolytes will help relieve constipation. Movement and exercise can also help reduce the constipated effects of fasting.

How Does Fasting Affect My Chronic Condition?

Fasting affects chronic conditions in many ways. One of the most significant ways in which fasting affects chronic disease is by increasing autophagy. Increased autophagy leads to increased cellular regeneration. This means that damaged cells are replaced while your immune system gets a break and can become stronger. Furthermore, your body enters a state of cellular protection and regeneration. This increases your body's response to stress and can help reduce the risk and severity of chronic disease. Your specific chronic disease may also determine how fasting works to improve your diagnosis and reduce the symptoms of that disease.

Fasting has proven beneficial for most chronic diseases, including Alzheimer's, cancer, heart disease, stroke, irritable bowel syndrome, SIBO, stroke, arthritis, diabetes, and more. Your chronic disease type will determine the best and safest fasting protocol to follow. While certain chronic diseases may take longer to show improvement with fasting, you can also combine fasting with other lifestyle and dietary changes for improved results. Regardless of the chronic disease you have, fasting will likely have a positive effect on your diagnosis.

Is Prolonged Fasting Dangerous?

Prolonged fasting is risky, especially if you don't follow the correct protocols. If you are pregnant, breastfeeding, underweight, or currently taking certain medications, prolonged fasting may lead to unwanted side effects. In this case, it is better to consider other therapy options for your chronic disease. Furthermore, you should never combine prolonged fasting with dry fasting as you may become dehydrated, and your health could suffer as a result. Ensure you drink plenty of fluids and electrolytes during a prolonged fast. Electrolyte imbalances may lead to health complications, specifically complications with your heart, which is why you should maintain proper electrolyte levels while fasting.

Another risk of prolonged fasting is refeeding syndrome after concluding the fast. Re feeding syndrome can lead to electrolyte imbalances, which may affect your heart. Furthermore, it can cause digestive distress, leading to diarrhea, nausea, vomiting, or constipation. Therefore, it's important to reintroduce food slowly when breaking a prolonged fast and to get plenty of rest.

Can I Eat During Prolonged Fasting?

While you can strictly eat foods that are less than 500 calories and contain no sugars or carbs without obstructing your body's fasting process, most experts recommend avoiding food, especially solid food, as far as possible while fasting. Instead, you can drink herbal tea, plain coffee, water, and electrolytes. In certain cases, you can also enjoy some vegetable soup (fewer than 500 calories). The foods you are permitted to eat will depend on your fasting plan. For example, if you are at a fasting clinic, they may provide certain approved meals prepared by the clinic's chefs that won't break your fast.

If you want to include solid foods in your prolonged fasting routine, I would recommend discussing the matter with a nutritionist first. Sticking to the liquids discussed earlier in this book will give you the best results during a prolonged fast. Your body will get all the nutrients it needs, so you won't need to eat solid foods during this time. Considering some of the other practices, such as meditation and exercise, can distract you while fasting, helping to reduce your hunger pangs and how often you think of food.

Can Fasting Heal My Cancer?

Fasting has shown great benefits for preventing and treating cancer. While there is currently no cure for cancer, fasting has many proven benefits for cancer prevention and treatment. Fasting prevents cancer by reducing your blood sugar levels, which puts your body in a state of ketosis. While it focuses on burning fat for energy, your immune system is strengthened, and your body produces several hormones that can help protect your body against inflammation and chronic disease. Furthermore, fasting prevents and combats cancer by putting your healthy cells in a state of protection and regeneration.

While your healthy cells learn to survive the stress of fasting, cancer cells don't have the same ability. In fact, they require constant food, specifically sugars, to multiply and grow. Therefore, by reducing your blood glucose levels and increasing your healthy cells' resistance to stress, prolonged fasting can essentially starve the cancer cells while keeping your body healthy. This is also useful for keeping your body healthy during chemotherapy. Fasting can increase your body's resistance to chemo toxicity, making the cancer cells more vulnerable.

Can Fasting Heal My Diabetes?

Fasting can heal type-2 diabetes and may provide relief from type-1 diabetes as well. As mentioned in the previous section, prolonged fasting reduces blood glucose levels. If you stop eating, your body processes all the sugars in your blood, stabilizing your blood glucose and insulin levels. This can prevent insulin spikes, which reduces your risk of developing diabetes. It can also reduce your blood glucose levels, reduce your risk of type-2 diabetes, and may cure it. The longer you fast, the more your blood glucose levels will stabilize, and your insulin levels will, too, as a result.

Furthermore, prolonged fasting can also heal and prevent diabetes by reducing your body fat percentage. When you fast, your body uses stored fat for energy. This reduces your body fat percentage, which helps you lose weight and maintain a healthy body weight. This also helps reduce insulin spikes, which can reduce and prevent diabetes. Combining fasting and healthy eating habits, such as a ketogenic diet or a low-carb diet, can help improve your health and heal your diabetes condition. Furthermore, these habits can prevent diabetes from occurring, which makes fasting a great preventative measure if you have been diagnosed with an increased risk of diabetes.

Can Fasting Heal My IBS?

Fasting is not only beneficial for cancer and diabetes. It can also improve your gut health and heal IBS. Irritable bowel syndrome often arises as the result of inflammation in the body. Poor lifestyle choices can also increase your risk of IBS, as can food allergies or intolerances. Fortunately, fasting has significantly increased your gut health and can heal your IBS. Fasting reduces inflammation by relieving the stress on your central nervous system. Fasting can also help your gut restore during fasting by giving your digestive system a break. This allows your gut flora to replenish and can restore your gut health.

Furthermore, fasting can heal IBS by strengthening your immune system. A strong immune system is crucial for improved gut health and reduced inflammation. Therefore, by enhancing your immune system, fasting can reduce IBS symptoms and heal your gut. Of course, it is also important to incorporate gut-healthy foods during your eating windows to heal IBS and improve gut health. These foods include healthy fats, fermented foods, and lean proteins. This can also improve your gut health and may reduce IBS symptoms and other symptoms of digestive distress.

Can Fasting Heal My Heart Problems?

Fasting can heal several heart conditions, including angina, arrhythmias, and progressive heart failure. Fasting can also decrease your risk of heart attack, which is a growing concern for many. Fasting can improve your heart health by managing your weight. Obesity is a common cause of certain heart conditions, and fasting can reduce your body fat percentage. Fasting can also heal heart problems by reducing inflammation in the body. Some heart conditions are caused by inflammation, especially those caused by inflammation, such as inflammatory heart disease.

Furthermore, fasting can improve your overall health, which may also improve your heart health. By reducing blood pressure, LDL cholesterol, inflammation, and stress, fasting can help your heart in many ways. Again, you can improve your heart health even more by combining fasting with other healthy lifestyle choices, such as moderate exercise, good quality sleep, healthy eating habits, and more. Drinking enough water and including electrolytes in your diet can improve your heart health, prevent heart disease, and heal existing heart conditions.

Can Fasting Reduce Damage Caused by Stroke?

Fasting is not only beneficial for improving your health and preventing disease. It can also be used to promote recovery after injury. For example, fasting has been shown to help reduce the damage caused by stroke. As mentioned before, fasting improves autophagy, increasing cellular regeneration and repair. Furthermore, fasting reduces inflammation and improves your body's immune system, which helps prevent secondary infections. By reducing inflammation, fasting can lead to improved healing. Fasting may, therefore, increase your healing time.

Fasting may also increase the quality of your healing after a stroke. In the second book of this series, we discovered that fasting improves neurogenesis, which is the brain's connection to the body. By increasing neurogenesis, fasting can help restore the connections that may have been damaged during the stroke, restoring the brain to its previous condition. As such, fasting can not only repair the damage caused by a stroke but might actually help to improve the longer-lasting fasting effects.

Can Fasting Reduce Damage Caused by Heart Attack?

Just like fasting can reduce damage caused by a stroke, it can also reduce the damage caused by a heart attack. During a heart attack, many of the fibers and vessels in your heart are put under immense strain and can sustain permanent damage as a result. Following a heart attack, you may have a weakened heart, and your blood flow may be compromised as a result. However, fasting can help to reduce the effects of a heart attack on your overall health and may help you recover faster. By reducing inflammation and increasing cellular repair, fasting can help your heart recover after a heart attack much faster.

Fasting can lead to angiogenesis, which promotes the growth of blood vessels in the body. This can also improve your heart's condition and help it recover from a heart attack. Fasting can help prevent further complications from a heart attack, such as secondary infections. By focusing on protection and recovery, your body gives your heart everything needed to recover and grow strong again. By incorporating fasting and other healthy lifestyle techniques, you can ensure your heart remains strong and healthy for many years.

How Long Can I Fast for My Chronic Condition?

As you can likely already tell from the previous chapters, there isn't really a specific period of time recommended for prolonged fasting. Some people prefer to do frequent

72-hour fasts, while others commit to a 21-day fast upon being diagnosed with a chronic disease. You may think that the longer, the better, but that is not always the case, especially not for a prolonged fast if you have had no prior fasting experience. Instead, it is recommended that you consider your specific chronic disease and what you want to accomplish when determining how long you plan to fast. If you want to do an extended fast, such as the ones mentioned in this book, you may consider doing so at a fasting clinic where your health is monitored.

If not, it is crucial that you follow the correct fasting protocols. They include drinking enough water and electrolytes, ensuring good quality sleep, and focusing on recovery while fasting. By doing so, you will give your body everything it needs to effectively use the time you are fasting to improve your chronic disease. If prolonged fasting seems too daunting, you can also start with a shorter, more manageable fasting model and increase the intensity from there.

Key Takeaway From Chapter 11

This chapter gave you insight into many of the frequently asked questions about fasting and chronic disease. While these were just shortened answers to the questions, you can find the extended explanations for these questions in the previous chapters of this book, as well as the previous two books in this series.

Chapter 12:

The Future of Chronic Diseases—The Case of Cancer

Before we end this book, I would like to share more information that can really help cancer patients in their quest for a cure. Alternative therapies are not discussed often enough as a cancer treatment, and many doctors (with the best intentions) focus on chemotherapy, radiation, and surgery. However, as you may have noticed in this book, there is another way. We discussed the impressive and promising effects of fasting on cancer, but there is also one more factor to consider. That is the idea that cancer is a metabolic disease and can be abolished if treated as such. One of the leading doctors in this field is Professor Thomas Seyfried, who has made significant advancements in the field of cancer as a metabolic disease.

In an interview with Dr. Eric Berg, Professor Seyfried explained that the primary difference between normal cells and cancer cells is that normal cells require oxygen to get energy and grow. In contrast, cancer cells use a fermentation process that does not require as much oxygen to grow. Instead, cancer cells require sugar and protein (glutamine) to grow and develop (Berg, 2018a). Professor Seyfried has studied the metabolic structure and function of cancer cells for many years and has determined that cancer can effectively be combatted if it is starved of its metabolic fuel.

Based on his research, Professor Seyfried deduced that you need to attack cancer cells on two fronts. You must remove its energy sources, namely glucose (sugar) and glutamine (protein). As you already know, a ketogenic diet can manage glucose. Cancer cells cannot utilize ketones for energy like healthy cells can. So, by adopting a ketogenic diet, you are starving the cancer cells of one fuel source. The other front on which to attack cancer cells is by inhibiting glutamine in the body. Here, Professor Seyfried has explored the use of DON, which is a glutamine-inhibiting drug. This drug was first developed in the 1950s and is considered a chemotherapy drug.

Professor Seyfried mentioned in his interview with Dr. Berg that they have not encountered or developed a drug more powerful at inhibiting glutamine at this point (Berg, 2018a). Therefore, by implementing a ketogenic diet to starve the cancer cells of glucose and using DON to starve the cells of glutamine, you are essentially removing the cancer cells' fuel sources. Not only does this prevent them from growing further, but it will also cause them to starve. According to Professor Seyfried, no known type of cancer could survive an environment without glutamine or glucose. Therefore, combining these two principles (ketogenic diet and DON therapy) can effectively cure cancer.

Unfortunately, Professor Seyfried explains that this therapy is not currently used in cancer clinics or treatment centers, so thousands of people still die from the disease. Many researchers are solely focused on the genetic component of cancer, so they don't consider other cancer-causing factors and are therefore not exploring all treatment options. Therefore, this treatment option is not currently being explored to its fullest extent. At this point, the hope is that the more exposure Professor Seyfried's work gets, the likelier this cancer treatment may become. This therapy may save millions of people in the future and already saves hundreds of people globally.

This is wonderful news. It could mean a cure for cancer. And if you have been diagnosed with cancer recently, I implore you to read Professor Seyfried's book, *Cancer as a Metabolic Disease*, and equip yourself with the necessary knowledge, discuss this treatment option with your oncologist and determine how you can starve the cancer cells of their fuel source—it might just save your life. Hopefully, the medical field will catch up with the science soon, and we will see this treatment plan being implemented to save patients worldwide. The more this type of research is discussed and awareness increases, the more interest in these therapies will grow. Funding will increase, and the treatments will finally be used to treat and cure patients.

While this specific therapy is regarding cancer, you have seen the effects of fasting and other alternative therapies throughout this book. Hopefully, these therapies will gain some traction in the future to cure cancer and other debilitating chronic diseases.

Keeping the Flame Alive

You now have the tools to take charge of your health and manage your chronic condition with the power of fasting. It's time to share that light and show others where they can find the same support.

Simply by leaving your honest thoughts about this book on Amazon, you'll be a beacon for others searching for answers. You'll help pass the knowledge in *Fasting Secrets for Chronic Conditions* forward, igniting hope and possibility.

Thank you for being a part of this journey. The conversation about using fasting to improve health keeps going when we share what we know—and you're helping me do exactly that.

Tina Shelton

Conclusion

Congratulations on finishing the book! Hopefully, you have learned much in these 12 chapters and now know how to take your health to the next level. This book was packed with useful information regarding fasting and chronic disease and how to implement fasting protocols to overcome your disease. Whether you have cancer, heart disease, or diabetes, this book has shared all the tips and necessary tools for implementing fasting to overcome chronic disease.

We started this book by explaining what a body without chronic disease looks like so you know what to look forward to when treating your condition. We then explained some of the most common chronic diseases, including heart disease, stroke, diabetes, cancer, and autoimmune diseases. We discovered how these diseases are identified, diagnosed, and treated. We then discovered different fasting models and explained how fasting works, its effects on your body, and some general benefits of fasting. That chapter gave you a better idea of all your fasting options and which ones may benefit your chronic disease most.

Thereafter, we focused on prolonged fasting. While shorter fasting models will offer some benefits for chronic diseases, prolonged fasting enhances all those benefits to really give you an effective treatment plan. We considered the risks, benefits, and hacks for making prolonged fasting effortless. We also discussed who should not attempt prolonged fasting and which precautions to take when prolonged fasting. After that, we discussed how to correctly break a prolonged fast. Incorrectly doing so can lead to several side effects and health problems. We discussed the importance of certain vitamins and minerals while fasting and how to conclude a prolonged fast safely. Then, we considered the body's nutrition systems when fasting. We also discussed the importance of electrolytes when fasting.

We considered how to incorporate prolonged fasting and fast-mimicking to treat and prevent certain chronic conditions, namely cancer, heart disease, stroke, diabetes, and IBS. We then considered the scientific evidence for fasting and chronic disease, shared some of the primary studies used throughout this book, and considered how research may develop in the future. In Chapter 9, we shared the actionable steps you can take to improve your health with fasting. We considered the tools you can use to improve your health and well-being while fasting, and we considered which biohacks you can incorporate to increase the effects of fasting on your health.

Case studies that demonstrate just how effective prolonged fasting, intermittent fasting, and the ketogenic diet are for treating and overcoming chronic disease were considered. These case studies serve as an inspiration for what you can achieve using the actionable steps and fasting protocols in this book. We then answered some of the frequently asked questions about fasting and chronic disease. Finally, we considered new research and studies that may offer a cure for cancer, and how important it is to spread awareness of these therapies.

Now that you have all the information, actionable steps, and science-based facts, all that is left is for you to implement what you have learned in this book. Consider the best fasting protocols to implement in your life, and how you can combine fasting with certain eating practices for increased health. Remember to consider your fasting goals when choosing a fasting plan and ensure that the plan is sustainable. Start slow and see how your health gradually increases and how your chronic disease disappears.

Glossary

Angina: A symptom of coronary artery disease. Angina is a term used to describe the type of chest pain associated with heart disease, such as tightness in the chest, difficulty breathing or squeezing in the chest.

Angiogenesis: The formation of new blood vessels. Angiogenesis occurs naturally in the body and increases during fasting. This process involves the growth, migration, and differentiation of endothelial cells.

Apoptosis: A biochemical event that occurs naturally in the body and leads to "cell suicide." Certain cells, such as cancer cells and certain types of yeast that are perceived as a threat by the body, experience Apoptosis because of the changes the body causes in those cells. This is your body's way of dealing with cancerous cells by itself.

Aspergillosis: An illness caused by a mold/fungus of the same name. If mold spores are inhaled, aspergillosis can lead to airway infections in people with weakened immune systems. It may lead to coughing blood, shortness of breath, and other health problems.

Benign: A benign tumor does not cause cancer in the body. It can be a lump of grown cells that are not cancerous. Benign tumors are usually removed surgically, and a diagnosis is often confirmed after removal.

Carcinogens: These are substances or factors that are known to increase your risk of cancer. There are many types of carcinogens, including environmental, physical, chemical, and biological. Despite knowing of the potential cancer-causing effects of some substances, companies are still allowed to use many carcinogens in their products.

Cardiovascular System: Consists of the heart, arteries, veins, and capillaries. The cardiovascular system pumps oxygen-rich blood to the body and removes oxygen-poor blood from organs.

Congenital Heart Disease: This is a problem with your heart that has been there since birth. Some people with congenital heart diseases can live for many years, even for life. In other cases, the problem will worsen and will eventually require fixing.

Diastolic Blood Pressure: The pressure in your arteries between heartbeats (when your heart rests). Diastolic blood pressure is one of the measurements used to determine heart health.

DNA: Deoxyribonucleic acid is the genetic roadmap to all organisms. Each person and creature has a unique DNA sequence, and the genetic code in DNA determines all organisms' growth, development, functioning, and reproductive potential.

Endocrine: The endocrine system consists of your lymph nodes, part of your brain, your reproductive organs, and anywhere else where hormones are produced. The endocrine system is responsible for hormone production and function throughout the body.

Gestational Diabetes: This is a type of diabetes pregnant women sometimes get. It may put the fetus at risk but usually disappears once the baby is born. Gestational diabetes is quite common and is caused by the fetus's strain on a woman's body during pregnancy.

Exertional Dyspnea: Feeling an intense shortness of breath or like you cannot fill your lungs with air. This is a common side effect of several heart conditions, including heart failure.

Ghrelin: The hormone responsible for making you feel hungry.

Growth Differentiator Factor (GDF): GDF describes a group of proteins that are primarily secreted and used during a growth phase. For example, children have higher GDF counts as they require more growth potential.

Herpes: This is a type of virus that causes blisters and ulcers. It is extremely common and can be found around the mouth and nose (HSV1) or around the genitals (HSV2). The herpes simplex virus is chronic and cannot be cured, though it can lay dormant for many years.

High-density Lipoproteins (HDL): Known as "good cholesterol." HDL helps regulate and remove excess

LDL cholesterol. Having higher HDL levels is a sign of good health.

HSC: Hematopoietic Stem Cells are the blood and marrow cells produced in the bone marrow. These cells are vital for a healthy immune system and fighting the effects of aging and chemo toxicity.

Hypokalemia: A condition during which your blood potassium levels are too low. Hypokalemia can occur when your electrolyte levels are imbalanced and may result in abnormal heart rhythms.

IBS: Inflammatory bowel disease is an umbrella term that describes various conditions that cause chronic bowels and digestive tract inflammation. IBS can lead to ulcers forming along the large intestine, small intestine, and colon. It can interrupt nutrient absorption and may lead to leaky gut syndrome.

IGF-1: Insulin-like Growth Hormone is a hormone that is produced by the liver. It functions just like HGH. While IGF-1 is crucial for tissue growth and fat mobilization during fasting, it has been linked with cancer, as it is a growth hormone and also prohibits Apoptosis.

Insulin: A hormone secreted by the pancreas to manage glucose that enters the bloodstream after you have eaten.

Korsakoff Syndrome: A chronic disorder that affects your memory. It is caused by a thiamine deficiency and is often associated with alcohol use over a long period.

Leptin: The hormone responsible for making you feel full.

Low-density Lipoproteins (LDL): Known as "bad cholesterol." If your LDL levels are too high, you may be at risk for cardiovascular diseases or stroke.

Low-GI: Foods with a low glycemic index are slower to release their glucose, causing fewer glucose spikes and, therefore, fewer insulin spikes after eating them. They are a better alternative to processed foods, leading to higher insulin spikes. Low GI foods include wholegrain pasta, wholegrain bread, brown rice, and sweet potato.

Malignant: Malignant means evil or malicious. A malignant tumor has been caused by cancer and can continue to spread cancer cells throughout the body, causing the cancer to spread.

Mormon: An American Christian religion based on the Church of the Latter-Day Saints. The Mormon church was founded in America in 1830 by Joseph Smith.

Osmosis: The exchange of materials from a high water content to a lower water content through a permeable membrane. Osmosis occurs between cells in the body and helps keep the body hydrated while removing waste products from cells.

RNA: Ribonucleic acid is found in living organisms and is responsible for most biological functions. While DNA is double-stranded to form a helix pattern, RNA is a single-stranded structure.

Ribosomes: These structures are made up of RNA and protein. It is where protein synthesis occurs in the cell and instructs the mRNA structures to create certain proteins.

Systolic Blood Pressure: The pressure in your arteries when your heart pumps. Systolic blood pressure is also used to determine heart health.

Telomere Length: This indicates how quickly your body (and cells) age. The longer your telomere length, the slower your body is aging.

Thiamine: Also known as vitamin B1, thiamine is an important vitamin for brain health. A thiamine deficiency can lead to memory loss and other central nervous system conditions.

Wernicke's Encephalopathy: A life-threatening disease associated with confusion, ophthalmoparesis with nystagmus, and ataxia. It is caused by the depletion of thiamine in the brain and may cause death.

References

About chronic diseases. (2022). Centers for Disease Control and Prevention. https://www.cdc.gov/chronicdisease/about/index.htm

Aitkon-Young, K. (n.d.). *The Beginner's Guide to Intermittent Fasting.* IBS Game Changer. https://www.ibsgamechanger.com/blog/intermittent-fasting-for-ibs

Ajmera, R. (2023, February 28). *The 4 Stages Of Fasting & Their Benefits: An Hour-By-Hour Breakdown.* Mindbodygreen. https://www.mindbodygreen.com/articles/stages-of-fasting

Angiogenesis Inhibitors. (2018, May 1). National Cancer Institute. https://www.cancer.gov/about-cancer/treatment/types/immunotherapy/angiogenesis-inhibitors-fact-sheet

Bais, L. (2023, April 19). *Intermittent Fasting vs. Prolonged Fasting: Differences, Pros and Cons.* BOXROX. https://www.boxrox.com/intermittent-fasting-vs-prolonged-fasting-differences-pros-and-cons/

Berg, E. (2013). The Myth about Blood Sugars and Diabetes [YouTube Video]. In *YouTube.* https://www.youtube.com/watch?v=P7fHYSy vxU0

Berg, E. (2018a). Discussion on Cancer with Professor Thomas Seyfried – Dr. Berg's Skype Interview [Youtube Video]. In *Dr. Eric Berg DC.* https://www.youtube.com/watch?v=Yyt3Do4 w7fs

Berg, E. (2018b, August 9). *Fasting: Miracle-Gro For Brain – Dr.Berg.* Www.youtube.com. https://www.youtube.com/watch?v=2-VhEwCziKA

Berg, E. (2018c, September 5). *What Does EDTA Do? – Dr. Berg.* Dr. Eric Berg DC; Youtube. https://www.youtube.com/watch?v=sFH-0Uu24-c

Berg, E. (2018d, October 22). *Refeeding Dangers After Prolonged Fasting - Dr.Berg On Refeeding Syndrome.* Dr. Eric Berg DC; Youtube. https://www.youtube.com/watch?v=9V8xMm kTf64

Berg, E. (2021a, November 24). *The Fasting Drink List: Dr. Berg's Guide to What You Can Drink During Fasting.* Dr. Eric Berg DC; Youtube. https://www.youtube.com/watch?v=v0lrJXU9 2-Q

Berg, E. (2021b). Why Does the Middle East Have the Lowest Cancer Rates in the World - Dr. Berg. In *www.youtube.com*.
https://www.youtube.com/watch?v=539UQ-6wC3g

Berg, E. (2022a, January 9). *The 5 BIG Prolonged Fasting Mistakes: MUST WATCH*. Dr. Eric Berg DC; Youtube.
https://www.youtube.com/watch?v=j9c6zkXr9U4

Berg, E. (2022b). From Stage 3 Colon Cancer to NO Cancer Detected in 4 Months. In *YouTube*.
https://www.youtube.com/watch?v=YzPrxku1x5Y

Bhardwaj, N. (2021, January 22). *Did you know walking barefoot on grass can improve your health? These 5 benefits are proof!* Healthshots.
https://www.healthshots.com/preventive-care/self-care/5-surprising-benefits-of-walking-barefoot-on-grass/

Can Fasting Prevent Strokes and Aid Stroke Recovery? (2019, May 30). Zero.
https://zerolongevity.com/blog/can-fasting-prevent-strokes-and-aid-stroke-recovery/

Cellular Health: What Is It And Why Is It Important? (2023, March 24). Www.next-Health.com. https://www.next-health.com/post/cellular-health-what-is-it-and-why-is-it-important

Chatterjee, R. (2023). What Happens After 30 Days of COLD SHOWERS? - This Will SHOCK YOU! | Dr. Susanna Søberg [Youtube Video]. In *Dr. Rangan Chatterjee.* https://www.youtube.com/watch?v=5udactTA 5IY

Chelluboina, B., Mehta, S. L., Chokkalla, A. K., Bathula, S., Park, J. S., & Vemuganti, R. (2020). Abstract WP138: Intermittent Fasting Prevents Ischemic Progression and Promotes Long-Term Recovery. *Stroke,* *51*(Suppl_1). https://doi.org/10.1161/str.51.suppl_1.wp138

Cheng, C.-W., Adams, Gregor B., Perin, L., Wei, M., Zhou, X., Lam, Ben S., Da Sacco, S., Mirisola, M., Quinn, David I., Dorff, Tanya B., Kopchick, John J., & Longo, Valter D. (2014). Prolonged Fasting Reduces IGF-1/PKA to Promote Hematopoietic-Stem-Cell-Based Regeneration and Reverse Immunosuppression. *Cell Stem Cell,* *14*(6), 810–823. https://doi.org/10.1016/j.stem.2014.04.014

Chronic Disease. (n.d.). Physiopedia. https://www.physio-pedia.com/Chronic_Disease

Chronic Disease Risk Factors. (2010). Public Health Agency of Canada. https://www.canada.ca/en/public-health/services/chronic-diseases/chronic-disease-risk-factors.html

Chronic illness. (2012). Better Health Channel. https://www.betterhealth.vic.gov.au/health/he althyliving/chronic-illness

de Toledo, F. W. (2022, August 19). *Benefits of long-term fasting with Dr. Françoise Wilhelmi de Toledo.* Buchinger Wilhelmi Clinic I the Fasting Experts; Youtube. https://www.youtube.com/watch?v=wYjWYCl _120

Doctor O'Donovan. (2022). Doctor explains INTERMITTENT FASTING for weight loss + METHODS and 10 FOODS TO EAT AND AVOID! In *YouTube.* https://www.youtube.com/watch?v=ahnl7GaV _rU

Eldridge, L. (2023, June 8). *Can Air Fryers Cause Cancer?* Verywell Health. https://www.verywellhealth.com/can-air-fryers-cause-cancer-5082537

Electrolytes for Fasting. (n.d.). Hydrant. https://www.drinkhydrant.com/blogs/news/el ectrolytes-for-fasting

Fasting and Chronic Illness. (2020, November 19). The Institute for Functional Medicine. https://www.ifm.org/news-insights/fasting-chronic-illness/

Fasting Electrolytes. (n.d.). Nutri-Align. https://www.nutri-align.com/fasting-electrolytes/

Fluck, D., Fry, C. H., Gulli, G., Affley, B., Robin, J., Kakar, P., Sharma, P., & Han, T. S. (2023). Adverse stroke outcomes amongst UK ethnic minorities: a multi-centre registry-based cohort study of acute stroke. *Neurological Sciences: Official Journal of the Italian Neurological Society and of the Italian Society of Clinical Neurophysiology, 44*(6), 2071–2080. https://doi.org/10.1007/s10072-023-06640-z

Gajagowni, S., Tarun, T., Dorairajan, S., & Chockalingam, A. (2022). First Report Of 50-Day Continuous Fasting in Symptomatic Multivessel Coronary Artery Disease and Heart Failure: Cardioprotection Through Natural Ketosis. *Missouri Medicine, 119*(3), 250–254. https://www.ncbi.nlm.nih.gov/pmc/articles/P MC9324723/

Geng, C. (2022, October 17). *Biohacking: What is it, types and hacks to try for beginners.* Medical News Today. https://www.medicalnewstoday.com/articles/biohacking

Gregor, M. (2023, January 19). *Podcast: Fasting and Cancer (Part I).* Nutrition Facts; Youtube. https://www.youtube.com/watch?v=9CxMsqpzhT4

Hamblin, J. (2019, March 13). *7 Biohacks That Actually Work.* The Atlantic. https://www.theatlantic.com/health/archive/2019/03/top-biohacks/584584/

Heavy Metal Poisoning (Heavy Metal Toxicity): Symptoms, Causes & Treatment. (2022, July 7). Cleveland Clinic. https://my.clevelandclinic.org/health/diseases/23424-heavy-metal-poisoning-toxicity

Henderson, E. (2023, March 7). *Long-term intermittent fasting can offer protection from heart-related COVID-19 complications.* News-Medical. https://www.news-medical.net/news/20230307/Long-term-intermittent-fasting-can-offer-protection-from-heart-related-COVID-19-complications.aspx

History of the company. (n.d.). Buchinger Wilhelmi. https://www.buchinger-wilhelmi.com/en/geschichte/

Integumentary System: What It Is, Function & Organs. (2022, April 25). Cleveland Clinic. https://my.clevelandclinic.org/health/body/22827-integumentary-system

Kharait, S. (2022, April 28). *Should you increase electrolyte intake during intermittent fasting.* Drink Magnak. https://drinkmagnak.com/should-you-increase-electrolytes-while-fasting/

Klimars, E. (2019, March). *This is what intermittent fasting does to your brain.* Radboud Universiteit. https://www.ru.nl/@1211513/what-intermittent-fasting-does-your-brain/

Lassila, L. (2021, January 30). *What Are The Benefits of Cold Showers?* BodyICE Australia. https://bodyice.com/blogs/all-things-bodyice/cold-showrs-for-recovery-fact-or-fiction

Learn about stroke. (n.d.). World Stroke Organization. https://www.world-stroke.org/world-stroke-day-campaign/why-stroke-matters/learn-about-stroke

Lindberg, S. (2019, March 27). *IBS Fasting: Benefits, Risks, Why It May or May Not Work.* Healthline. https://www.healthline.com/health/irritable-bowel-syndrome/ibs-fasting

Liu, Z., Liu, M., Jia, G., Li, J., Niu, L., Zhang, H., Qi, Y., Sun, H., Yan, L.-J., & Ma, J. (2023). Long-term intermittent fasting improves neurological function by promoting angiogenesis after cerebral ischemia via growth differentiation factor 11 signaling activation. *Plos One, 18*(3), e0282338. https://doi.org/10.1371/journal.pone.0282338

Longo, Valter D., & Mattson, Mark P. (2014). Fasting: Molecular Mechanisms and Clinical Applications. *Cell Metabolism, 19*(2), 181–192. https://doi.org/10.1016/j.cmet.2013.12.008

Lopez-Jimenez, F. (2022, October 8). *Wondering about fasting and heart health?* Mayo Clinic. https://www.mayoclinic.org/diseases-conditions/heart-disease/expert-answers/fasting-diet/faq-20058334

Mapson, A. (2023, June 4). *Ep.3 Intermittent fasting for IBS - When you should eat.* Goodness Me Nutrition. https://www.goodnessme-nutrition.com/podcast/intermittent-fasting-for-ibs-when-you-should-eat/

McIntosh, J. (2019, August 20). *Mold in the home: how big a health problem is it?* Medical News Today. https://www.medicalnewstoday.com/articles/2 88651

Mehanna, H. M., Moledina, J., & Travis, J. (2008). Refeeding syndrome: what it is, and how to prevent and treat it. *BMJ, 336*(7659), 1495–1498. https://doi.org/10.1136/bmj.a301

Michalsen, A., & Li, C. (2013). Fasting Therapy for Treating and Preventing Disease - Current State of Evidence. *Forschende Komplementärmedizin / Research in Complementary Medicine, 20*(6), 444–453. https://doi.org/10.1159/000357765

Mitchell, S. J., Bernier, M., Mattison, J. A., Aon, M. A., Kaiser, T. A., Anson, R. M., Ikeno, Y., Anderson, R. M., Ingram, D. K., & de Cabo, R. (2019). Daily Fasting Improves Health and Survival in Male Mice Independent of Diet Composition and Calories. *Cell Metabolism, 29*(1), 221-228.e3. https://doi.org/10.1016/j.cmet.2018.08.011

Nanehkaran, Y. A., Licai, Z., Chen, J., Zhongpan, Q., Xiaofeng, Y., Navaei, Y. D., & Einy, S. (2022). Diagnosis of Chronic Diseases Based on Patients' Health Records in IoT Healthcare Using the Recommender System. *Wireless Communications and Mobile Computing, 2022*, e5663001.
https://doi.org/10.1155/2022/5663001

Over the Hedge. (2006). IMDB. https://www.imdb.com/title/tt0327084/characters/nm0000246

Overview of the Endocrine System. (2015, July 6). United States Environmental Protection Agency. https://www.epa.gov/endocrine-disruption/overview-endocrine-system

Panoff, L. (2019, September 26). *What Breaks a Fast? Foods, Drinks, and Supplements.* Healthline. https://www.healthline.com/nutrition/what-breaks-a-fast

Patrick, R. (2016, October 1). *Valter Longo, Ph.D. on Fasting-Mimicking Diet & Fasting for Longevity, Cancer & Multiple Sclerosis.* Found My Fitness; Youtube.
https://www.youtube.com/watch?v=d6PyyatqJSE

Phillips, M. C. L. (2019). Fasting as a Therapy in Neurological Disease. *Nutrients*, *11*(10). https://doi.org/10.3390/nu11102501

Pizzino, G., Irrera, N., Cucinotta, M., Pallio, G., Mannino, F., Arcoraci, V., Squadrito, F., Altavilla, D., & Bitto, A. (2017). Oxidative Stress: Harms and Benefits for Human Health. *Oxidative Medicine and Cellular Longevity*, *2017*(8416763), 1–13. https://doi.org/10.1155/2017/8416763

Plez, M. (2023). PROVEN BENEFITS Of Prolonged Fasting: 3 Things That You Need To Know | Dr. Mindy Pelz [Youtube Video]. In *Dr. Mindy Plez.* Youtube. https://www.youtube.com/watch?v=i7YvR-7lKpc&t

A quote by Dr. Seuss. (n.d.). Www.goodreads.com. https://www.goodreads.com/quotes/7639135-when-something-bad-happens-you-have-three-choices-you-can

Ramos, M. (n.d.). *Intermittent Fasting: How to Break Your Fast.* Diet Doctor. https://www.dietdoctor.com/intermittent-fasting/how-to-break-your-fast

Rappaport, S. M. (2016). Genetic Factors Are Not the Major Causes of Chronic Diseases. *PLOS ONE*, *11*(4), e0154387. https://doi.org/10.1371/journal.pone.0154387

Regular fasting could lead to longer, healthier life. (2019, November 5). American Heart Association. https://www.heart.org/en/news/2019/11/25/regular-fasting-could-lead-to-longer-healthier-life

Roberts, H. (2022, February 1). *What healthy cholesterol levels should look like for you, explained in 2 charts.* Insider. https://www.insider.com/guides/health/conditions-symptoms/cholesterol-levels-by-age-chart

Rudolf Breuss Cancer Cure. (2023). Fasting.ws. https://www.fasting.ws/juice-fasting/cancer-treatments/rudolf-breuss-cancer-cure/

Sayer, A. (2023, June 13). *How To Break A Water Fast: 3 Helpful Tips.* Marathon Handbook. https://marathonhandbook.com/how-to-break-a-water-fast-3-helpful-tips/

Scheurlen, K. M., Billeter, A. T., O'Brien, S. J., & Galandiuk, S. (2020). Metabolic dysfunction and early-onset colorectal cancer – how macrophages build the bridge. *Cancer Medicine, 9*(18), 6679–6693. https://doi.org/10.1002/cam4.3315

Schuler, L. (2015, March 13). *This Guy Didn't Eat for 382 Days—and Didn't Poop for Almost 2 Months!* Men's Health. https://www.menshealth.com/health/a195337 28/craziest-diet-ever/

Seyfried, T. (2012). Cancer as a Metabolic Disease: On the Origin, Management, and Prevention of Cancer. In *Google Books*. John Wiley & Sons. https://www.google.co.za/books/edition/Canc er_as_a_Metabolic_Disease/4lrIjiL_hw8C?hl=e n&gbpv=1&printsec=frontcover

Seyfried, T. N., Flores, R. E., Poff, A. M., & D'Agostino, D. P. (2013). Cancer as a metabolic disease: implications for novel therapeutics. *Carcinogenesis*, *35*(3), 515–527. https://doi.org/10.1093/carcin/bgt480

Sherrell, Z. (2023, February 24). *Cancer-causing foods.* Medical News Today. https://www.medicalnewstoday.com/articles/c ancer-causing-foods

Should You Drink Electrolytes While Fasting? | My Own Water. (2022, November 26). My Own Water. https://www.myownwater.com/blog/benefits-of-electrolytes-while-fasting

Shrimanker , I., & Bhattarai , S. (2021, July 26). *Electrolytes.* Pub Med. https://pubmed.ncbi.nlm.nih.gov/31082167

Sissons, C. (2020, May 27). *What percentage of the human body is water?* Medicalnewstoday. https://www.medicalnewstoday.com/articles/what-percentage-of-the-human-body-is-water

6 cold shower benefits to consider. (2023, January 25). UCLA Health. https://www.uclahealth.org/news/6-cold-shower-benefits-consider

Stanislaw, J. (2022, December 14). *Intermittent fasting and type 1 diabetes?* Dr. Jody Stanislaw; Youtube. https://www.youtube.com/watch?v=8RXUi53 5kUA

The Statistics of IBS: How Many People Suffer from the Condition? (n.d.). GI Associates. https://gi.md/test-colonoscopy/the-statistics-of-ibs-how-many-people-suffer-from-the-condition

The story of Angus Barbieri, who went 382 days without eating. (2018). Diabetes. https://www.diabetes.co.uk/blog/2018/02/story-angus-barbieri-went-382-days-without-eating/

TEDx Talks. (2019). Intermittent Fasting: Transformational Technique | Cynthia Thurlow | TEDxGreenville. In *YouTube*. https://www.youtube.com/watch?v=A6Dkt7z yImk

Time to try intermittent fasting? (2020, July 1). Harvard Health. https://www.health.harvard.edu/heart-health/time-to-try-intermittent-fasting

Trochon, J. J. (2021, January 7). *My book*. Jean-Jacques Trochon. https://jeanjacquestrochon.com/my-book/

Understanding acute and chronic inflammation. (2020, April 1). Harvard Health. https://www.health.harvard.edu/staying-healthy/understanding-acute-and-chronic-inflammation

Valayer, S., Kim, D., Fogtman, A., Straube, U., Winnard, A., Caplan, N., Green, D. A., Flora, & Weber, T. (2020). The Potential of Fasting and Caloric Restriction to Mitigate Radiation Damage—A Systematic Review. *Frontiers in Nutrition, 7.* https://doi.org/10.3389/fnut.2020.584543

Wang, Y., & Wu, R. (2022). The Effect of Fasting on Human Metabolism and Psychological Health. *Disease Markers, 2022,* 1–7. https://doi.org/10.1155/2022/5653739

Wegman, M. P., Guo, M. H., Bennion, D. M., Shankar, M. N., Chrzanowski, S. M., Goldberg, L. A., Xu, J., Williams, T. A., Lu, X., Hsu, S. I., Anton, S. D., Leeuwenburgh, C., & Brantly, M. L. (2015). Practicality of Intermittent Fasting in Humans and its Effect on Oxidative Stress and Genes Related to Aging and Metabolism. *Rejuvenation Research*, *18*(2), 162–172. https://doi.org/10.1089/rej.2014.1624

Weinsier, R. L. (1971). Fasting—A review with emphasis on the electrolytes. *The American Journal of Medicine*, *50*(2), 233–240. https://doi.org/10.1016/0002-9343(71)90152-5

What Are the Health Benefits of Consuming EDTA? (2015, June 16). Livestrong; Youtube. https://www.youtube.com/watch?v=XYZvCp DrEXM

Wilhelmi de Toledo, F., Grundler, F., Bergouignan, A., Drinda, S., & Michalsen, A. (2019). Safety, health improvement and well-being during a 4 to 21-day fasting period in an observational study including 1422 subjects. *PLOS ONE*, *14*(1), e0209353. https://doi.org/10.1371/journal.pone.0209353

Wilhelmi de ToledoF. (2022, February 10). *Dr Françoise Wilhelmi de Toledo : L'art de jeûner.* Métamorphose, Éveille Ta Conscience; Youtube. https://www.youtube.com/watch?v=rZYOIH_2aUQ

Wilhelmi, B. (2021a, January 18). *How to prepare the perfect fasting soup? | All about fasting Q&A.* Buchiner Wilhelmi Clinic; Youtube. https://www.youtube.com/watch?v=pv4aiV5Qpxo

Wilhelmi, B. (2021b, February 5). *The Benefits of Long-term Fasting.* Buchinger Wilhelmi Clinic - the Fasting Exerperts; Youtube. https://www.youtube.com/watch?v=rPL8QSng2sY

Wilhelmi, B. (2021c, February 19). *The Buchinger Wilhelmi Fasting Protocol l Buchinger Wilhelmi.* Buchinger Wilhelmi Clinic - the Fasting Experts; Youtube. https://www.youtube.com/watch?v=z90cUXq9DqU

Worldwide cancer data. (n.d.). World Cancer Research Fund International. https://www.wcrf.org/cancer-trends/worldwide-cancer-data

Wu, S. (2014, June 5). *Fasting triggers stem cell regeneration of damaged, old immune system.* USC News. https://news.usc.edu/63669/fasting-triggers-stem-cell-regeneration-of-damaged-old-immune-system/

Printed in Great Britain
by Amazon